Resolving Grievances in the Nursing Home

COLUMBIA UNIVERSITY SCHOOL OF SOCIAL WORK
COLUMBIA STUDIES OF SOCIAL GERONTOLOGY AND AGING
SOCIAL WORK AND SOCIAL ISSUES

RESOLVING GRIEVANCES
in the
NURSING HOME

A Study of the Ombudsman Program

ABRAHAM MONK
LENARD W. KAYE
HOWARD LITWIN

Columbia University Press
New York • 1984

Library of Congress Cataloging in Publication Data
Monk, Abraham.
Resolving grievances in the nursing home.
(Social work and social issues)
Bibliography: p.
Includes index.
1. Nursing homes—United States—Complaints against.
2. Ombudsman—United States. 3. Nursing homes—Law
and legislation—United States. 4. Nursing home
patients—Legal status, laws, etc.—United States.
I. Kaye, Lenard W. II. Litwin, Howard. III. Title.
IV. Series. [DNLM: 1. Nursing homes—Standards—United
States. 2. Patient advocacy. 3. Homes for the aged—
Standards—United States. WT 27 AA1M7r]
RA997.M65 1983 362.1'6'068 83-7606
ISBN 0-231-05702-4

Columbia University Press
New York Guildford, Surrey

*Clothbound editions of Columbia University Press books are
Smyth-sewn and printed on permanent and durable acid-free paper.*

Dedicated to the memory of
Hyman J. Weiner *and* **Charles Grosser**
teachers, mentors, friends

CONTENTS

PREFACE

As the authors of this study of nursing home ombudsmen note, the dramatic increase in the numbers of very old adults (the seventy-five-year and older cohort) has resulted in an explosion of long-term care facilities. Further, federal labor force statistics project gerontological social work as the second of ten major growth industries in the 1990s (just behind industrial robot production!). The current and projected expansion of programs for the aged attests to the timeliness of this work, but timeliness is one of its lesser virtues. The study is important on a number of counts; I shall cite three.

For one, the book may well foreshadow a direction of advocacy in the 1980s. It provides an overview of the literature on mediation and advocacy and summarizes information on the principles of ombudsmanship as applied in several social contexts as well as in the field of aging. Thus, although its focus is on how the concept works in long-term care, the usefulness of the study transcends that field. Through its documentation of how a publicly supported program can mobilize community responsibility to enhance the protection of vulnerable citizens, the study implicitly highlights the role of government in assuring quality services, even in these days of regressive social policy. The ombudsman concept reflects a commitment to opening institutions (such as long-term care settings) to scrutiny and to direct communication between the community, service provider, and consumers of service (in this instance, the elderly). In part too, the study sheds some light on the interesting question of whether "organizational troublemakers" may not indeed serve the functions of organizations by forcing adjustments which make them more viable entities. Not that the success of the ombudsman as advocate is by any means overstated; for success is, in fact, limited. Apparently, the intervention of an ombudsman is more beneficial to individual residents of homes then as a source of policy change. Nevertheless, the authors demonstrate that ombudsmen and advocates serve as significant humanizing elements in institutional care.

Another virtue of the study is its willingness to let the data speak for itself. The book eschews polemics and sidesteps the heat and turbulence of the nursing home debate. In so doing, it illuminates the complexity of the environment in which the institutional aged find themselves. As might be expected, views on public accountability, health care, patients' rights, and the quality of life in nursing homes differ sharply among the participants in the system. The study reports these divergent views with precision and objectivity but without editorial comment, although there are implications to be drawn from them. For example, the authors define three major roles assumed by ombudsmen: mediator, advocate, and therapeutic supporter, and explore the impact of the respondents' location within the long-term care network on their views of the appropriateness of one or another role. Clearly, ombudsmen are influenced in their choice of role not by who they are as much as by their organization's function, structure, and constraints. What is less apparent is whether the ombudsmen are aware of the extent to which these factors influence their views and performance. Exposure to the systematically collected perspectives of the multitude of actors in the health care system constitutes a major benefit of the study, and is likely to increase the understanding of a wide variety of publics regarding service provision in the field, such as health care advocates, policy-makers, program planners, administrators, and long-term care service workers.

A third, and perhaps more important contribution of this study is the connection it makes between empirical research and practical program alternatives or policy directions. For example, the authors cull from their data the programmatic consequences of particular choices that have been made in the process of developing ombudsman programs and the ways in which the decisions governing their selection determine outcome. Their description of these various pathways provide important direction to those who would now establish programs. Too often the collection of data is not similarly transformed by researchers into workable material that is useful to practitioners. In this case the translation from "numbers to words" has been successfully maneuvered without detriment to analytical precision. The process is intriguing and a case in point for those who would seek to better guarantee the practical utility of survey research.

From my perhaps biased perspective as a social welfare administrator, one set of findings in the study is striking. In these days in which profit-making and the workings of the market are viewed in some powerful quarters as the most effective and efficient bases for structuring social services, the study is illuminating. The authors have discovered that residents of proprietary homes rate the quality of care lower than their peers in nonprofit facilities. Furthermore, clients in proprietary homes fear staff retaliation, if they turn to an ombudsman, to a greater degree than those in voluntary settings, and they therefore complain less than their peers. The combination of poorer quality of care and more limited freedom to complain in the proprietary homes is a finding that is suggestive in the profit vs. nonprofit controversy, and, it is to be hoped, of use to national policy makers. At the least, it is a finding that those who are concerned about the future status of the elderly in American society will find important.

But then, there are numbers of significant findings in this study, and they are perhaps best left to unfold for themselves in the pages that follow.

George Brager
Dean, Columbia University School of
Social Work

ACKNOWLEDGMENTS

The idea of conducting a study of nursing home ombudsman programs was first formulated during the winter and spring of 1979. The Community Council of Greater New York had implemented a nursing home patient ombudsman program in New York City one year earlier with funding from the New York City Department for the Aging and the New York State Office for the Aging. The Council readily provided sanction and encouragement for the development of the research proposal which was subsequently submitted to the American Association of Retired Persons (AARP) Andrus Foundation. A second-stage study of state ombudsman programs situated throughout the United States came to be a natural outgrowth of this initial local investigation. Phase II was presumed to afford us an opportunity to determine the extent of similarities and differences between local-level and state-level patient mediation in long-stay facilities.

Survey research, whether limited to a locality or extending across the nation, necessarily involves the contributions of numerous individuals and organizations. The authors wish to acknowledge those without whose cooperation and assistance this study could not have been successfully carried out.

The study would not have been possible without the continuing financial support over a two-year period from the American Association of Retired Persons Andrus Foundation. We are indebted to the Foundation's board of trustees, its chairman at the time of the study, Olaf J. Kaasa, and Frederick J. Ferris, the Foundation administrator, and his staff. An additional grant from the Charles and Lois Silberman Fund and the Columbia University School of Social Work made possible the transformation of the original technical reports into book form. Additional thanks are due John D. Moore and Charles Webel at Columbia University Press.

Bernard Shiffman, executive director of the Community Council, and Sylvia Hunter, former director of the New York City nursing home ombudsman program, provided initial encouragement for the research endeavor. Hunter's successor, Patricia M. Belanger, and her staff were most cooperative in providing access and local program information throughout the course of the New York City study.

Numerous members of the Columbia University community were also instrumental in enabling the execution of the study. In particular, Mitchell I. Ginsberg, former dean of the faculty, George Brager, dean of the faculty, and Muriel Reed, assistant dean and director of admissions of the Columbia University School of Social Work.

We also benefited from the advice and guidance of: Sue Wheaton and Anne Hart, Long Term Care Ombudsman Program, Office of Program Development, Administration on Aging; Barbara Frank, National Citizens' Coalition for Nursing Home Reform; Anne Trueblood, American Association of Homes for the Aging; Karen Comeaux, New York State Long Term Care Ombudsman Program; and countless other legal, medical, and social welfare professionals functioning in the long-term care network.

Staff and consultants at the Brookdale Institute on Aging and Adult Human Development at Columbia University provided editorial, administrative, technical, and moral support throughout the course of the study. They included Karin Bradford, Maida Rosenstein, and Carl Brenden. Dr. Brenden deserves a special note of thanks for his expert performance of data processing and statistical functions. L. R. Hults processed early drafts and the final computerized manuscript.

Various Columbia University and Barnard College student interns warrant acknowledgment for their contributions in the areas of field interviewing, secondary analysis, and questionnaire coding: Susan Alberts, Joe David Garner, Jr., Thomas Glover, Ruth Hershenov, Carol Hunt, Onnie Lovett, Francine Rubin, Barbara Tobey, Robert Townley, and Cheryl Turner.

Finally, our inestimable gratitude has been earned by the numerous individuals who, in the interest of contributing to improved care for nursing home residents, gave of their time to respond to our investigative probes. We thank the many ombudsmen who graciously allowed us to visit and observe their state programs as well as the various groups of survey respondents who voluntarily and thoughtfully replied to the survey questionnaires.

Of course, the authors themselves bear full responsibility for the interpretations and conclusions contained within this book.

Resolving Grievances in the Nursing Home

Introduction

This book presents the findings of a study on ombudsman services for the aged in long-term care facilities. The research was aimed at determining the extent to which volunteer and federally sponsored advocacy programs have succeeded in introducing a system of community involvement and public scrutiny of the services older persons receive in long-term care settings, commonly designated "nursing homes." The study was focused, for the most part, on the ombudsman as agent for complaint resolution, and it assessed the degree to which such individuals, whether public officials or volunteers, can correct and eventually reverse abusive or neglectful treatment of frail elderly residents in long-stay institutions.

The great increase in the use of nursing homes or long-term care facilities constitutes one of the major developments in health care policies and services in the last two decades. The need for such facilities, far from abating, will sharply expand in the future as the number of elderly in general, and more specially those over age 75, continues to rise. There were 12 million older persons in 1950, 25 million in 1980, and the number will reach the 45-million-level by the year 2000.[1] The cohort aged 75 and older however, is growing at a faster pace than any other age segment in the American population. In 1976 they constituted 38 percent of the 65+ age group. Their proportion will reach 45 percent by the year 2000. In absolute terms, it will double in the last quarter of this century from 8 million to 15 to 19 million.[2]

Prevalence of chronic disabilities, a leading cause of institutionalization, similarly rises with age. Serious limitation in the capacity to carry on major activities more than doubles in the population aged 85 and older as compared to the cohort 65 to 74 years of age, from 14 percent in the latter group to 31 percent in the older one.[3] Need for assistance to carry out basic tasks of daily living such as dressing is nine times higher among the group 85 and older than among those 65 to 74 years of age: 18 percent of the former require such help compared to only 2 percent in the younger cohort. Moreover, while only 2 percent of the 65 to 74 years-old group requires assistance with bathing and only one percent with toileting, among those age 85 and older these needs climb to 11 percent and 7 percent, respectively.[4] Dependency-inducing disabilities augment with age, and even if they can be controlled or delayed by advances in rehabilitative treatment, decreases in mortality rates are bound ultimately to increase morbidity rates. In other words, as more people survive into their 70s and 80s, more individuals will require assistance and for longer periods of time. Use of nursing homes by age groups confirms this assertion: in 1977 there were about 13 nursing home residents per 1,000 persons age 65–74; there were 216 nursing home residents per 1,000 persons age 85 years and older.[5]

Millions of Americans have resorted to nursing home care in recent years. Their number climbed, in fact, by 302 percent between 1960 and 1976, from 331,000 to 1,327,300.[6] The quality of the care they received, however, has been repeatedly denounced for its proclivity to abuse and insensitivity to human needs.

Abuse and Victimization of Patients

A fifteen-year study by the Senate Special Committee on Aging, published in 1974, concluded that "at least half of the nation's nursing homes have one or more serious, life threatening conditions."[7] Documented hazards range from the neglect of daily life amenities to theft, poor food, the deliberate infliction of physical injuries, unsanitary conditions, overmedication, adverse drug reactions, frequent medication errors, and the possibility of death by fire.[8] A policy analysis by Vladeck indicates, furthermore, that such effects are not aberrations but rather the natural extension of a policy of rational cost minimization.[9] The evidence of abuse and the recognition of its roots in public health policy led Vladeck to recommend that nursing homes be opened to outsiders, such as volunteers, to provide the vigilance that the system requires.

In a pioneer study calling attention to the deplorable living conditions of nursing homes during the 1950s, Jules Henry focused on the residents' sense of degradation and hopelessness. He characterized nursing homes as "pathogenic" institutions liable to transform their patients into children or robots, in a way similar to that in which psychiatric institutions "animalize" their patients.[10]

Henry's extreme conclusions are contradicted in a more recent ethnographic study by Kayser-Jones, which points to possible cultural determinants of nursing home deficiencies.[11] Comparing two such institutions, one in Scotland and the other in the United States, Kayser-Jones found residents in the former more independent and more satisfied in a seemingly "homelike environment." Their American counterparts were, however, more despondent, unhappy, enjoyed less freedom, and lived within a constraining and austere environment.

Searching for the root of these negative conditions, Bennett, Pincus, and Kosberg and Tobin alluded to the standardized rewards and punishments and regimented, fixed routines in nursing homes in terms reminiscent of Goffman's analysis of total institutions.[12] Coe, and Lieberman, Tobin, and Slover, found, however, marked differences in the degree of totality and potential harmful consequences of the nursing homes under scrutiny.[13] Sectarian, voluntary, and nonprofit facilities stood out more positively than proprietary ones in terms of quality and individuation of care.

Stannard and Blumenthal et al. cite the poor training and lack of incentives for aides and paraprofessionals—those who work most closely with the patients—as the leading explanation of the problems under review.[14] Far from identifying themselves with the therapeutic objectives of their places of employment, aides were seen to lose all motivation, to become cynical about the possibility of achieving any results, and to concentrate their energies on the more manageable goals of maintenance and custody. When they cannot control their charges, their only recourse within a limited repertoire of skills is the abuse of authority. Management and professional staff are restrained in attempts to root out abuse because aides are difficult to recruit, given their minimal wages. Moreover, their high turnover rates disrupt any semblance of uniformity and continuity of care. The resulting vicious circle is obvious and hard to break.

Picking up the trail left by the literature on total institutions of the preceding two decades, Kayser-Jones systematized the most frequently reported problems in nursing homes into four categories:

1. *Infantilization.* This includes the scolding, patronizing, and rewarding of older persons as if they were irresponsible, dependent, even if likable children.
2. *Depersonalization.* Patients are treated as "nonpersons," as if they do not exist, or do not count, the end result being the loss of individuality and attachment to one's lifelong social system. Depersonalization occurs through:
   (a) *Symbolic means,* when patients' pleas for help are ignored and staff avoids communicating with them
   (b) *Routinized care,* when patients are cared for in assembly-line fashion, given no choices, and denied a say in anything pertaining to their care or amenities
   (c) *Lack of protection,* when basic health needs are provided tardily and with ill will, or go unattended, thus threatening the person's physical survival.
3. *Dehumanization.* This is a more deleterious and extreme form of depersonalization, in which the person is not only humiliated and debased, but also denied the treatment naturally expected in human service settings: understanding, respect, compassion. This

includes situations such as exposing genitals, bathing men and women together, and forcing patients to urinate in public.

4. *Victimization.* In this phenomenon theft of patients' possessions is denied by the institution. Such refusal to accept responsibility adds insult to the patient, who in many instances is blamed for "imagining" the alleged losses. Victimization also encompasses punitive restraints, sedation, and verbal abuse or intimidation.

Kayser-Jones concludes that "if one lives in a society that does not value the aged, it becomes easy to victimize that group, and the institutionalized aged, a weakened and dependent group, become 'captive victims' for predators."[15]

Corrective Strategies

The search for amelioratives to this "sordid record of exploitation," as characterized by a July 15, 1982 New York *Times* editorial, has followed the growth of nursing homes. A score of corrective strategies and resources, many of which can be activated by the institutionalized aged themselves, have evolved in recent years.[16] Included among these are public interest legislation, advocacy interest groups, associations comprised of friends and relatives, laws dealing with abuse of patients, and nursing home patient ombudsman programs. Nevertheless, the limited success of statutory and regulatory efforts outside the nursing home to monitor patients' care complaints successfully has been well documented.[17] At the same time, the call to initiate alternative long-term care monitoring strategies, such as nursing home ombudsman programs, has been discussed at more frequent intervals.

Anderson found that the characteristics of the nursing home are consistent with the ombudsman approach.[18] He described the nursing home structure as approximating a rational bureaucracy in which staff, nurses, orderlies, and administrators work in a hierarchical framework of delegated authority, a chain of command. The addition of an ombudsman to mediate between the links in the chain, therefore, may well be seen by all as beneficial. Furthermore, society bears a special obligation to make sure that the services provided for its institutionalized elderly are indeed satisfactory.

An alternate way of reaching a positive conclusion concerning the nursing home ombudsman is to document that other methods of regulation simply do not work. Regan noted that there are three such approaches: establishing national standards for the facilities, instituting an adequate reimbursement formula, and promoting quality care through professional standards review organizations (PSROs).[19]

Donabedian, in relating to the first of these methods, challenged the assumption that the provision of a certain environmental standard leads to good medical care.[20] Critics of the method, furthermore, view legal standards as a national farce. Regan noted for example that despite established standards, government "rarely decertifies facilities or seeks criminal sanctions for non-compliance."[21] Weatherby also denounced the failure of enforcement devices and the failure of standards.[22]

The second method assumes that adequate care will follow from sufficient expenditures. Regan observed an alternate result in which the health facility simply produces higher priced care and higher profit margins with the increase in available funds. Wildavsky has termed this phenomenon "The Law of Medical Money," noting its appearance in many facets of the health industry.[23]

The PSRO, the third alternative, has been variously termed "a government plea for medical involvement in the effective and efficient distribution of medical services," or "the first major intrusion of government into the private delivery of health care."[24] Encompassing aspects of utilization review and peer review, the PSRO is designed to assure that necessary services are adequate and economical, through self-regulation of organized medicine. The mechanism is problematic, however.

First, it is hampered by "dependence on acceptance by physician groups" on the one hand, and by "the unwillingness of professional groups to impose punitive sanctions on their own members."[25] Second, it suffers from excessive bureaucratization, and third, in regard to the long-term care facility, what is to be reviewed by the PSRO may be "subjective, judgmental and unquantifiable."[26] Decker and Bonner confirm that "the state of the art of nursing home evaluation is far less developed than the evaluation of hospital care.[27] Thus, in light of these developments, adoption of a nursing home ombudsman may be seen as a desirable option.

Public Policy and the Ombudsman

The initial implementation of the nursing home ombudsman may be traced to seven demonstration projects established through the U.S. Department of Health, Education, and Welfare in 1972 and 1973. Forman's analysis of the program shows varied application of the ombudsman concept, ranging from an almost traditional, legislatively founded ombudsman in Massachusetts, to the establishment of state and local units that focused upon the use of trained senior citizen volunteers.[28] The findings from the experience as reflected in several unpublished state reports indicate that the nursing home ombudsmen saw their role as actively advocating the rights of the elderly and in bringing about broad systemic reforms through new legislation and new facility regulation. The use of volunteers, on the other hand, was not viewed enthusiastically, particularly because of the extended effort required to train them. As Regan sums up, "the partisan position recommended for the office in these reports [was] inconsistent with the neutrality traditionally associated with an ombudsman."[29]

The demonstration projects were followed by a change in the programs' funding, administration, and direction. The Administration on Aging (AoA), under the directives of the Older Americans Act amendments of 1975, set up yearly grants to most of the states to appoint an ombudsman development specialist, and to spur "the development of voluntary community action groups as the new ingredient in the process of settling complaints of nursing home patients."[30] The focus shifted to the organization of an ombudsman process, in contradiction to the demonstration projects' recommendations. Regan noted the fears of excessive cost, questionable effectiveness, and the political unpopularity of a patient advocacy emphasis. Delany and Davies document just such a case in Pennsylvania where the state legislature made renewed funding conditional upon the cessation of litigational activity by the nursing home ombudsman office.[31]

The 1978 amendments to the Older Americans Act and the rules and regulations attached to these amendments continued in only partially addressing the recommendations derived from the experiences of the original ombudsman demonstrations.[32] Thus state agencies on aging were assigned the responsibility of establishing and operating statewide long-term care ombudsman programs. Operations could be carried out directly by each state or through contracts with any public or private nonprofit organization. Long-term care facilities are defined broadly in the regulations and include skilled nursing facilities, intermediate facilities, nursing homes, and other adult care homes. Requirements concerning access to facilities, residents, and patients' records; confidentiality; disclosure of records and files; and the establishment of a state-wide uniform reporting system to collect and analyze information on complaints and conditions in long-term care facilities were more vaguely defined. Furthermore, the regulations stipulated that each state must use annually one percent of the state allotment for social services or $20,000, whichever is greater, to operate the long-term care ombudsman program. Only American Samoa, Guam, the Virgin Islands, the Trust Territory of the Pacific Islands, and the Northern Mariana Islands are not subject to the above expenditure requirements.

The Primary Support Networks Alternative

The ombudsman program was a product of the 1970s, a decade of heightened and zealous concern with patients' rights.

The program must be seen as part of a broader movement that sought to bolster the professionalization and accountability of long-term care services. Stringent controls and regulations were the inevitable corollary of the public outrage with nursing home conditions, but as Barney observed, ordinary regulatory mechanisms do not work with services which have disabled, powerless people as their clientele. Unless external pressure is relentlessly exerted, service agencies will forgo the primary imperative of high-quality care and respond instead to the more immediate concerns for efficiency and profitability. Barney continued arguing for a community presence, with anyone coming in regularly to nursing homes—volunteers, relatives, and friends—keeping up the pressure and the warning that "someone out there" really cares.[33]

Gottesman and Bourestom confirmed that there is a strong relationship between the rate of visitors and good care,[34] but since many nursing homes' residents do not have relatives and receive visits very infrequently, a federal ombudsman program is viewed as the only supportive resource left to which residents may turn.

Curiously, the 1980s are witnessing a growing movement aiming to restore the primacy of the so-called "natural support networks" in the provision of care for the elderly. Although a noble aspiration, it is hardly a realistic one. Families and friends can play a significnt role in such care, but they are not in a position to deal with the multiple requirements of their aged kin and acquaintances for prolonged and indefinite periods of disability. There are, indeed, families whose solicitous care reaches the limits of self-sacrifice. Moreover, the idealization of the primary supports alternative often rests on the argument that families already provide 85 percent of the home health care services for older relatives.

Families do fill many gaps and deficiences of the service system, far beyond household chores. Some family members even take courses to learn how to perform complex rehabilitative tasks. There is reason to wonder, however, how much maintenance the average family can provide beyond basic socioemotional support and essential chores, and for how long. Eggert et al. reported that families' ability or willingness to continue home care services drops by 50 percent after the second hospitalization of their disabled elderly relative.[35] The average family is not insensitive, but the extent of its capacity to provide care is not infinite, either. In any event, the primary support networks of nursing home residents are weakened or may have alrady disintegrated. Moss and Halamandaris point out that the average age of nursing home residents is 82, and only one in ten has a living spouse. Two thirds are widowed, and one in five were never married. Moreover, over 50 percent have no living relatives, and 60 percent receive no visitors.[36] For this population, nursing homes will remain the arrangement of necessity. Doing away with these facilities clearly constitutes a misguided and harmful policy aspiration. It is far more positive to try to do something about the care they provide. The ombudsman program is a step in that direction.

Conclusion

Nursing home patient ombudsman programs are a recently estabished component within the gerontological service continuum. They were created with the expectation of improving the lines of communication among families, community, and residential institutions. While sanctioning the continuation of nursing home ombudsman programs, however, the 1978 Older Americans Act legislative mandate remains vague and allows for considerable variation in the types of interventive efforts implemented by separate state and regional programs. Similarly, a review of applications of the ombudsman concept in this and other fields of service renders a confusing picture of a disparate array of interventive functions or role behaviors, all of which are defined as essential components of this redress mechanism. Clearly, no definitive resolution techniques have yet emerged. In the absence of well-defined policy that could provide such programs with ample legislative authority and more precisely defined objectives, it becomes especially important to examine the ways in which nonstatutory empowerment strategies serve as policy substitutes.

Having introduced the problem under scrutiny, this book proceeds to review the historical, philosophical, and political antecedents of the ombudsman idea. It will then examine where the ombudsman program fits in the present constellation of quality control and regulatory mechanisms in the human services field. This is the content of chapters 1 and 2, which serve as the conceptual background for the empirical report of the ombudsman study. Chapter 3 describes how the study evolved as well as its methodology and implementation. Chapters 4, 5, and 6 present the major findings, and chapter 7 attends to the program's continuity and the conditions necessary to render it more effective in the future.

CHAPTER ONE
Antecedents of the Ombudsman Program

Until the mid 1960s the office of ombudsman was a little known phenomenon in the United States, and relatively little was written about the few ombudsmen who then functioned in the countries of northern Europe. The mid and late 1960s, however, saw a major reversal of this situation. With the publication of what are now considered classic comparative studies[1] and the subsequent importation of the ombudsman role into varying and sundry realms of American public life, the office became a much sought after, if still little understood, administrative ameliorative. Indeed, the United States was said to have become engulfed in "Ombudsmania."[2]

The proliferation of papers on the ombudsman and its ubiquitous application did not, nevertheless, result in a clear delineation of the role, structure, and function of that office, nor of the appropriate form its adoption in American society should assume. Even today, the efficacy of the ombudsman mechanism remains an area of considerable controversy. Interpretations of the office have ranged from the most limited kind of administrative intervention, usually in the form of a recommendation for redress, to visions of the ombudsman as a "cure-all."[3]

The range of institutions and levels of public administration in which the ombudsman was instituted similarly revealed the lack of a central conception of the role and its function. This multiplicity of meanings of "ombudsman" portended that "the word will be preserved without any defined content, that any suggested Mr. Fix-it with or without ascertainable authority or function will be accorded the name ombudsman."[4] Indeed, "the ombudsman concept is still in a formative stage in this country; its ultimate role in our society remains to be determined."[5]

The following pages trace the evolution of the ombudsman concept in its varying applications, noting especially the diversity of role, structure, and function that the position has embodied in its respective forms, as well as its subsequent adoption in the human services system. Regan's distinction between classical, executive, and hybrid forms of the ombudsman serves as a useful yet tentative classification along which to organize the discussion of the ombudsman literature.[6] In addition, a comparison of the ombudsman role with that of another type of mediating agent, the advocate, underlines both similarities and dissimilarities in the conceptual parameters of these two intervention strategies.

The Classical Ombudsman

The classical ombudsman type is most closely approximated by the Scandinavian countries' application of the office. Perhaps it is more accurate to say that since they were the first countries to implement the ombudsman (Sweden 1809; Finland 1919; Denmark 1955; Norway 1962) the form the office took there became subsequently known as the "classical" type. Whatever the case, as Rowat indicates, even among the Scandinavian countries "significant variations exist . . . in their arrangement for protecting citizens against arbitrary authority."[7] It would seem, therefore, that the classical ombudsman can serve as an ideal type for the sake of analytic comparison rather than as a necessarily accurate denominator of the phenomenon itself.

Various attempts have been made to identify the universal components of the classical ombudsman type. Rowat isolated three essential features embedded in the classical definition:

1. The ombudsman is an independent and nonpartisan officer of the legislature, usually provided for in the constitution, who supervises its administration.
2. He deals with specific complaints from the public against administrative injustice and maladministration.
3. He has the power to investigate, criticize and publicize, but not to reverse, administrative action.[8]

Gellhorn, a pioneer in the study of ombudsmen, details the differences among respective ombudsmen in his comparative study of nine nations. He notes, nevertheless, that there exist common strands as well. The following characteristics constitute somewhat of a common denominator for classical ombudsmen: expertise (usually legal training), selection by legislative bodies, independence (subject to periodic renewal), response to complaints *or* self-initiation of inquiry, periodic inspection of governmental establishment, explanatory decisions, and the power (but not the preference) to recommend or order prosecution.[9]

Hill has written extensively on the position of the New Zealand ombudsman which, like its Scandinavian counterparts, is formulated along classical lines. Established in 1962, "the New Zealand institution has become the primary model for the world's newer ombudsmen."[10] Unlike the Scandinavian precedent, however, the holder of the New Zealand office is "the first ombudsman appointed in a common law jurisdiction,"[11] thus demonstrating the successful adaptation of the concept to nontraditional surroundings.

Hill makes the effort, based upon his New Zealand research, to develop a more comprehensive definition. He isolates the following characteristics of the classical ombudsman: (1) legally established; (2) functionally autonomous; (3) external to the administration; (4) operationally independent of both the legislature and the executive; (5) specialist; (6) expert; (7) nonpartisan; (8) normatively universalistic; (9) client-centered but not antiadministration; and (10) both popularly accessible and visible.[12]

Moore examines the application of the ombudsman idea to a nonclassical situation, in this case to the antipoverty programs of the 1960s, and notes the generic characteristics of the ombudsman: independent and impartial, expert, accessible, with power to investigate and to recommend but not revise.[13] His extrapolation of the ombudsman characteristics from the classical paradigms underlines the importance for the classical definition of the very characteristics that he did away with, namely, the sanction of the legislature and the supervisory focus on public administration. Thus in their absence in Moore's discussion, the legislative and governmental variables reflect an inherent association with the classical ombudsman concept.

That is not to say that every legislative sanction is functional for the classical definition. The British Parliamentary Commissioner for Administration (PCA), appointed in 1967, is a case in point. The British PCA deals with complaints only after they have been filtered through ministers of Parliament. Thus the ombudsman of the British Parliament is not empowered to investigate on his own initiative.[14]

In his comparative survey, Stacey found the British ombudsman to be relatively inaccessible.[15] The difficulty of access in combination with the exclusion of numerous administrative sectors from his jurisdiction is a significant diversion from the "ombudsman ideal." The parliamentary connection, therefore, seems to provide the British PCA with more limited scope instead of greater independence, suggesting that what has been created is not an ombudsman but rather, in Gwyn's words, an "ombudsmouse." Indeed, the negative reaction to the British ombudsman raises the possibility that deviation from the classical model may have dysfunctional consequences. Dolan notes this possibility as fact, writing that anything other than the classical version is not worth the time or the money it takes.[16]

The classical ombudsman role is intrinsically related to the existence of a national consensus. It is worth noting the conditions that foster consensus, therefore, and thus promote the success of the ombudsman mechanism. The Scandinavian countries and New Zealand are small, homogeneous societies, suggesting that public consensus may be more easily attained in such a context than in larger, pluralistic settings. In fact, concerning the applicability of the ombudsman, Anderson is quoted as noting that size is "the single most important factor in considering whether to transplant the institution to another country."[17]

Gellhorn's comment that the ombudsman is "most useful in a society already so well run that it could get along happily without his services at all" provides further insight into the necessary underlying conditions for the success of the office. It particularly cites a required lack of conflict in public administration. Linnane's review of the ombudsman observes that the aim of the office is to provide citizens with a sense of participation "in a government that is acting fairly."[18] Linnane thus reinforces the view that the classical ombudsman functions optimally in a consensus-oriented society. Indeed, the very purpose of the office would seem to be to strengthen popular consensus among the citizenry.

As crucial as the consensual framework is for the classical ombudsman, most conspicuous is its absence in the executive ombudsman type.

The Executive Ombudsman

In contrast to the classical ombudsman, Wyner defines the executive ombudsman as "a centralized complaint handling officer who has been appoined to office and who serves at the pleasure of an elected or appointed chief executive."[19] As such, both the ombudsman's power and his effectiveness are derived from the relationship with the chief executive who made the appointment. This is in sharp distinction from the independent classical type.

Following Wyner's comparison, Anderson outlines other significant differences between the two ombudsman models.[20] The executive ombudsman is seen as an active, result-oriented agent who strives to expedite government action. He is, therefore, often an initiator, unfettered by considerations of maintaining consensus among public officials. The classical ombudsman, on the other hand, is for the most part passive, usually acting subsequent to the receipt of complaints. He is more process-oriented, and his aim is most often directed at striving to streamline governmental procedure. The former may, in short, be seen to cut knots while the latter unravels red tape.

The problems that the classical ombudsman undertakes are consequently less urgent and not as likely to be "amenable to precipitous intervention" as those of his executive counterpart. Anderson places the differences of the two ombudsman models in perspective: the executive ombudsman exists to stimulate faster and better services while the classical ombudsman aims to stimulate the articulation of fair procedure in government. Clearly then, the role, structure, and function of each of the two types diverge significantly.

The question may be raised as to whether the executive ombudsman should indeed be called an ombudsman at all. Wyner points out that "formal titles are often misleading guides to actual task performance," while on the other hand "scores of American jurisdictions have created executive ombudsmen, many without ever hearing the term ombudsman."[21] In a similar vein, it may be seen that those states in the union which have adopted ombudsman mechanisms have shown significant divergence in the application of the term. Hill identified the Hawaiian ombudsman as the classical type. Anderson noted the developmental evolution of the Iowa Citizens' Aide Office from that of the executive to a full-fledged classical model. Oregon, on the other hand, chose to retain the executive model. The New Jersey Department of the Public Advocate, established in 1974, combined the legislative statutory independence of the classical model and the access to decision-making power of the executive model, while surpassing both models in its regulatory authority.[22]

Gwyn's study of the failure to implement a classical-type municipal ombudsman in Newark, New Jersey, outlines the

conditions under which the executive model may be preferable. Mayor Gibson sought to have his city included in the funds
offered by the Office of Economic Opportunity (OEO) for the
development of municipal ombudsmen. The mayor's approach to implementation of the project, however, epitomized
the contradiction between classical and executive ombudsman
types. When the mayor sought city council passage of the or-
dinance, as a classical model requires, the bill became associated with the mayor's own agenda and was thus opposed by
city council members hostile to their chief executive. The failure to gain consensus on the issue thwarted implementation
of the city ombudsman, and in the end the OEO funds were
returned to Washington unspent.

Gwyn commented after the fact that it was not at all clear
that such a classical ombudsman would have worked anyway:

> In retrospect, an ombudsman probably would not have succeeded in
> Newark. The city is so polarized, the political forces so diverse and mo-
> bilized, the bureaucracy so unresponsive, and the economic conditions
> so extreme, that an independent investigator of citizen complaints,
> backed by no political force of his own, would have been eaten alive in
> a matter of months.[23]

He concluded that whereas the implementation of a classical
ombudsman was impractical in Newark, the institutionalization of an executive ombudsman could have succeeded. Other
writers, however, have pointed to the weaknesses of the executive ombudsman as well. The use of the power of the chief
executive to enforce the ombudsman's stature may be seen as
a major shortcoming, exposing the ombudsman to charges of
bias and partiality as well as making his tenure uncertain.[24]

In the nonconsensual situations that are characteristically
addressed by the executive ombudsman, the ombudsman's
chief advantage, consensual persuasion, is ineffective. In such
cases more adversarial grievance mechanisms may be required. The hybrid type of ombudsman is often even more
distant from consensual persuasion than is the executive one,

and in certain cases has consequently adopted some of the very advocacy roles suggested for its executive counterpart.

The Hybrid Ombudsman

The hybrid ombudsman type presumes to respond to the dysfunction inherent in implementing the ombudsman function within large-scale, diverse settings. As Fitzharris spells out in a call for a corrections ombudsman, "the only realistic way to apply the ombudsman concept in a large state. . . . [is] by breaking the constituency down into specialty areas, such as corrections, mental health and welfare."[25] Representative of the hybrid ombudsman type, therefore, are various prison ombudsmen, university ombudsmen, and others in even less traditional areas. This section reviews a selected group of such ombudsmen, as reflected in the literature, in order to indicate the range and diversity of the concept's application in the recent past.

The Prison Ombudsman

A prime area in which a specialized ombudsman might be expected to be installed is that of prisons and corrections. In countries with national classical ombudsmen, prisoners' complaints generally make up about 10 percent of all citizen appeals.[26] In addition, as Stacey points out, the secrecy surrounding prisons emphasizes the importance of having available redress mechanisms for that class of facility.[27] Nevertheless, despite its apparent significance, the position of the corrections ombudsman is still a limited experiment in the United States, and there are varying opinions as to its efficacy.

Proponents of a prison ombudsman tend to associate the position with the classical nature of the function. Tibbles is one who envisions the corrections ombudsmen in such a traditional sense, stressing impartiality and the nonadversarial mode of functioning:

> He does not act in an adversary fashion, but remains independent of both the citizen and government as a mediator or intermediary. He attempts to see all sides of the dispute and bring a satisfactory resolution to the citizen's complaint.[28]

Cromwell similarly emphasizes the intermediary role and the power of persuasion:

> A jail ombudsman should have access to all inmates and should investigate all complaints which are not patently frivolous. Where, in his judgment, redress of grievances is warranted he should seek the assistance of the appropriate official who can remedy the situation.
> Many times the complaints of inmates stem from oversights and failures in communication. In these cases the ombudsman can simply bring the problem to the attention of the appropriate agency and have it corrected.
> These services should create an atmosphere in which the emotional strain of incarceration and the feeling of helplessness by the inmate is reduced to a minimum.[29]

While a number of states have correctional ombudsmen, only a few grant significant degrees of independence to them. Minnesota is one state that has created a bona fide ombudsman for corrections with sufficient independence and authority. In that state, the prison ombudsman is responsible solely to the governor, and as such constitutes an example of the "executive" version of the function. Despite the executive nature of his position, and his serving at the pleasure of the governor, the Minnesota corrections ombudsman nevertheless fills a role based on mutual cooperation and general consensus with the Department of Corrections, characteristics of the classical type.[30] The model that Fitzharris proposes in his call for a corrections ombudsman appears to approach the classical type exemplified by the state of Minnesota.[31]

Critics of the ombudsman idea in the domain of corrections have expressed reservations regarding the goal, function, and efficacy of the position. Anderson, Moore, and Cressey have taken a controversial position in this critical debate. They point out:

The prison ombudsman is different from all other ombudsmen because, no matter how you look at it or what he does, his entry in the prison results in the redistribution of power. . . . We want the prison to be unpleasant, and so we strip people of their power to make choices. In that kind of a setting the ombudsman represents a threat to the warden.[32]

They further cite as an obstacle the prison status quo of "echelon authority" within which one must seek to achieve a modicum of change. The ability of the ombudsman to do so is questioned as is the ombudsman's pliant form of entry into the prison, suggesting that it may come at the cost of acceding to the norms of the prison organization.[33]

Another criticism stems from the potential for prison ombudsmen to focus on individual cases only, and to refrain from considering their cumulative effects. Ombudsman survival may be achieved at the cost of avoiding recommendation of any systemic change. Furthermore, as the authors point out, "while ombudsman offices contribute to the incremental improvement of prisons, it is possible that they also thereby contribute to the overall maintenance of the status quo."[34] The implication of this concern would appear to surpass the specific reference to prison ombudsmen and leads to questioning the efficacy of the office in general.

The prison ombudsman adds new elements to the overall ombudsman concept. Among those may be counted the professionalization of the complaint-handling process, the fostering of improved communications in the facility, and the rehabilitative effect of moral suasion as opposed to force. Indeed, Anderson, Moore, and Cressey see this method of conflict resolution as "a maker of community in the prison."

Fitzharris also stresses the communication role that can help prevent rumors that lead to riots.[35] The Minnesota corrections ombudsman reported playing such a negotiating role that served to defuse a potential riot in the prison:

Crisis occurred three months after the ombudsman took office. The prison warden, the commissioner of corrections, and the prisoners requested his services to help negotiate the release of a hostage being held by three prisoners. In this instance, the ombudsman's role was to serve as a third and impartial party to the negotiations and to monitor the implementation of any negotiated agreement. After several hours of negotiation, the hostage was released unharmed, and the Department of Corrections did not have to make any unrealistic commitments. This incident identified the ombudsman as a resource in times of trouble for both the prisoners and the staff.[36]

Thus despite questions of long-term strategic effects, it has been variously reported that corrections ombudsmen may make an impact upon the quality of prison life, and may indeed effect improvements.

The Academic Ombudsman

Another area that appears to have adopted the ombudsman function on a large scale is that of academia. Over one hundred colleges had appointed ombudsmen by 1974.[37] Verkuil writes that "it may be that the university, or in a larger sense the school system, is the prototypical environment for the ombudsman in our society."[38]

It is Verkuil's contention that an ombudsman flourishes when he does not have to compete with the adversarial model. His thesis will be discussed later in this chapter, when comparing ombudsmanship with advocacy. For the moment, it is useful to note his conclusion: "The presence of the ombudsman may have the effect of restoring some of the sense of community, which is indispensable to the school system's ability to fulfill its crucial role in value formation."[39]

Numerous articles have appeared in the last decade in the area of university or school ombudsmen. Most are descriptive or prescriptive in nature, and subject to much leeway in their interpretations. Silverbank, for example, spells out the structural characteristics of the job of university ombudsman. She notes that such characteristics reflect "the organizational arrangements and climate of the particular institution." In her discussion, Silverbank specifically mentions that differences in the format the university ombudsman follows are contingent upon selection procedure, faculty, status, constituency, load credit allotted, and accessibility to alternate sources for settling disputes. Of particular interest from the point of view of this review is her observation that full-time university ombudsmen "tend to take a greater role in actively trying to restructure the bureaucratic system," while those who work part time "are content to solve individual problems."[40]

Silverbank thus characterized the job of the university ombudsman as liaison between students and the larger campus community. In another study, Grafton and Rivera similarly found that those students who used the services of a campus ombudsman perceived his role as that of an impartial mediator. Other writers, however, place more emphasis upon the role of ombudsman as guarantor of student rights.[41]

In an empirical study of the academic ombudsman, Stewart analyzed the treatment given a sample of complaints at a particular university. The data yielded two mutually exclusive ombudsman roles which he labeled respectively "conflict management" (serving the interests of the institution) and "conflict resolution" (client-centered advocacy geared toward systemic change). Stewart's study concluded that the university ombudsman tended to favor the role of conflict management, at the expense of conflict resolution.[42]

In a rebuttal to Stewart's conclusions, Harvey criticized the analysis as a reflection of the author's personal predilection for an advocacy or prosecutional ombudsman style.[43] She suggests that the reality is not so onesided, nor are ombudsman roles necessarily so mutually exclusive. Nevertheless, the debate over ombudsman style underscores the strategic dilemmas inherent in the ombudsman function. Does the ombudsman work only in situations of consensus, or are there roles that can include effective intervention in situations of dissension as well?

The range of role perceptions of the campus ombudsman gives some support to "the thought that each ombudsman must create and modify the role or function he or she plays while in office."[44] In addition, the conceptualization of conflict management versus conflict resolution styles, both of which are seen as legitimate, points out how far from the classical ombudsman model the university hybrid type has moved.

The Medical Ombudsman

The ombudsman in health service delivery and hospital settings shows even greater divergence from the office's classical roots. In particular, the juxtaposition of consensual versus conflict roles, as articulated in the debate on the ombudsman as a patient advocate, illustrates the widening parameters of perceptions held of the position.

It is useful initially to trace the relationship of the classical ombudsman to the field of health. Statements by the national ombudsman of New Zealand illustrate the case in point.

Hospital boards were first brought under the jurisdiction of the New Zealand ombudsman in 1968. This development opened the arena of debate on how to differentiate between administrative and professional decisions in health delivery. The ombudsman himself notes that "he must avoid straying into the area which properly belongs to the medical expert."[45] If any doubt remains, the New Zealand ombudsman further clarified that

> his function is not to reform the health system of the country or to improve the standard of medical care in particular institutions, but simply to determine whether a complaint should be sustained, and, if it can, to secure some redress.[46]

The hybrid-type ombudsman in health care delivery, on the other hand, tends to perceive his role quite differently from that of the classical ombudsman. Once again, the evidence is derived from descriptive and prescriptive reports, largely reporting on experiences in institutional settings.

Kopolow set the tone when he noted that the ombudsman's role is not to resolve individual complaints. Rather it is "to make recommendations to correct the system's malfunctioning." Madison similarly stressed the broader view of patients' rights which includes "identifying the gaps in health services affecting particular groups of patients or deficiencies in existing institutional services affecting the community as a whole."[47]

Broderick concurs with the reform role of the ombudsman in the health field and suggests that:

> The ombudsman's chief contribution may well be to identify those areas most pressingly in need of legislative attention, as well as those which can be performed from within by the particular administrative agency. . . . this function can best be carried out when limited to an isolated institution.[48]

He thus calls for the implementation of "a one-legged ombudsman," as he terms the hybrid type. Other studies have similarly noted the utility of ombudsmen as patients' advocates.[49]

There is less agreement, however, on how to put into operation the concept of the ombudsman as the patients' advocate. A call for the nurse to become a patients' advocate has been countered by inherent problems that suggest "someone other than the nurse . . . perform patient advocacy functions."[50] Katz has proposed that the ombudsman be a person on the outside unaffiliated in any other way with the institution. Kopolow suggests, on the other hand, a tripartite system composed of the patients' representative, a lawyer, and the ombudsman. Madison raises the strategic contradiction, namely, the lack of sanction which is placed in the hands of the patients' advocate, whose tools as ombudsman "are limited to moral suasion, tact, education and persistence." Perhaps in response to such strategic dilemmas, Robinson and Alboim suggest that the ombudsman role be carried out by young community representatives whose strong sense of commitment overcomes other potential limitations.[51]

Dissertations by Eckert and Mailick deal in varying degrees with the question of the ombudsman in health care. Eckert's study describes the ombudsman as an "archetypical advocacy mechanism." However, "without a rational public policy for the Health (Illness) Delivery System," and thus without the accompanying consensus in this area, "it is concluded that the ombudsman mechanism is non-efficacious."[52]

Mailick's study of patient-representative programs in short-term general hospitals saw the program in one sense as the institutionalization of an advocacy role.[53] She furthermore noted the relationship of the concept of ombudsman to that of advocacy. More significant, perhaps, is her observation that there are differences as well. The four types of programs that she conceptualized—grievance, personal service, financial service, and hospitality/information—reflect the differing roles that the representative (or ombudsman) may assume in different locations.

A final note needs be mentioned on the ombudsman role in noninstitutional mental health settings. Wolkon and Moriwaki reinterpret the ombudsman function as a primary prevention mechanism of psychological disorder. Their study of the KABC radio ombudsman in California found that the program provided "short term primary prevention by offering assistance to individuals in coping with external reality stresses." They conclude that the KABC ombudsman goes beyond the grievance process, gives the individual emotional support, and aids in developing a more adaptive approach to crises. A new role, therefore, that of therapist, is added to the repertoire of functions of the hybrid ombudsman.

> The ombudsman is handling problems with which, were there no ombudsman, the individual would be frustrated on a reality level and suffer on the emotional level. . . . It gives the individual emotional support through work with him to resolve his immediate problem and hopefully developing more adaptive approach to crises.[54]

The Social Welfare Ombudsman

The field of social welfare offers many opportunities to apply the ombudsman mechanism, but relatively little has been written about the experience of social workers as ombudsmen. A range of such possibilities that have been recorded include ombudsmen for the mentally retarded, welfare ombudsmen, and ombudsmen for such fields as crime and juvenile delinquency, mental illness, housing, and urban renewal.

In one of the few articles relating social work to ombudsmanship, the efficacy of the ombudsmanlike third-party role of expediter is prescribed for the social worker. In fact, the means and the ends of the two roles are seen to be similar. Payne suggests that:

> A social worker's potential contribution is obvious: his assistance in arbitrating disputes between social service institutions and their clients should enhance service and hopefully reduce the public scorn that such disputes frequently engender.[55]

An alternative view of the social worker as ombudsman becomes manifested in the legislative arenas. This role is aimed at compensating for the restrictions of the classical ombudsman type which concentrate, according to Zweig, on "how well a policy is carried out," rather than on "the desirability of the policy itself."[56] Zweig suggests, instead, instituting a social work policy ombudsman who would intervene at the level where policy is made.

Still another application of the ombudsman idea to the field of social welfare is reflected in Fox's call for an agency ombudsman, to humanize the accountability process. He notes:

> The most obvious area where the concept can be of use is to correct procedures, possibly arbitrary and capricious, of practitioners and administrators in both private and public agencies. . . . The role of ombudsman is constructed so as not to impinge or supplant, but to reinforce and supplement agency functions.[57]

Such calls avoid, however, the serious objections raised by some writers concerning the efficacy of the social worker as ombudsman. Hazard, for example, disputes the ability of the ombudsman to spur systemic change.[58] He views the lawyer as the professional more suited to defend individual case interests. To Hazard, "the power of the ombudsman is the power of suggestion," which does not have much motivating force in American society. Furthermore, social policy is so obviously repressive in his eyes that to discover evidence of this condition would not represent a needed service for the downtrodden. At the same time, however, he acknowledges the difficulty that OEO legal services experienced in attempting to turn case representation to class litigation, a dilemma which "helped excite interest in the idea of having an ombudsman" in the first place.

Cloward and Elman share Hazard's skepticism. They recognize that the ombudsman derives strength from a tradition of consensus, and for the very lack of such, they deem the position inappropriate for a welfare system (which in their view was designed to be unjust).[59] The welfare ombudsman would therefore be expected to fail "because his recommendations would run counter to public attitudes towards rights of the poor."[60]

Underlying the discussion of the social worker as ombudsman is a more basic differentiation that has been developed and discussed up to this point between ombudsman and advocate functions, the consensus and contest approaches, conflict management and conflict resolution, and so on. As presented in this discussion, the extension of the ombudsman concept into an executive and subsequently a hybrid format has blurred the boundaries of the position's very function, and has overlapped what have been formerly seen as exclusively advocacy functions. Later in the chapter, a selected review of literature will compare the two functions, ombudsmanship and advocacy. However, to complete the sketch of the evolution of the ombudsman, the next section traces some of the extremes to which the term has been applied.

A Range of Other Hybrid Ombudsmen

Mallory proposes an ombudsman for retarded and disabled people in residential institutions, a natural extension from the hospital setting, and an application similar to that of nursing home ombudsmen. Felton et al. apply the role to "new professionals," combining patients' advocate, integrator, and therapist functions. Their widened view of the role turns the ombudsman into a "mental health generalist." Pletcher, on the other hand, sees a specialized role, within the academic setting. He proposes the establishment of a curriculum ombudsman. Each of these proposals includes a minor variation which stretches the concept even further from its original image.[61]

The following role applications, however, apply the term ombudsman to situations so unlike the concept's structure and intention that one can only wonder at the lengths to which "ombudsmania" will yet be applied. Battle, for example, describes the pediatrician as ombudsman for young handicapped children. Koltveit views the school guidance counselor as a quasi-ombudsman. Nelson and Starck suggest the newspaper as ombudsman, while Smith and Winnick offer the library as ombudsman for the neighborhood.[62]

Finally, one even finds the extension of the concept into the realm of the family. Park and Shapiro suggest that parents should be ombudsmen for their own emotionally disturbed children. Milliken and Urich, on the other hand, propose the use of community ombudsmen to help parents recognize their children's difficulties at school.[63] Clearly, the hybrid ombudsman type has extended the boundaries of the concept far beyond the position's original purpose, to its potential advantage and perhaps to its detriment as well.

The Ombudsman and the Advocate

As a result of the occasional reference to the ombudsman as advocate, and the periodic interchanging of the two roles despite their reputed contradistinction, it is necessary to clarify the terms and their possible consequences. A review of the literature relating to this question reveals that while the labels are no longer mutually exclusive, there are underlying behaviors that remain apart. The following paragraphs spell out these differences, and their significance for the conceptualization of the ombudsman function.

The preceding pages traced the development of the definition of the ombudsman concept. It is necessary, therefore, to define briefly the term advocate for the sake of comparison.[64] Grosser observed that the role of advocate is taken, essentially, from the field of law. As such, the technique of advocacy embodies a role which is not one of enabler, broker, expert, consultant, guide, or social therapist. The advocate is, in fact, "a partisan in a social conflict, and his expertise is available exclusively to serve client interests."[65]

Grosser's later qualification, however, that the advocate makes "extensive use of collaborative and mediatory approaches," and "that adversarial strategies are generally appropriate only as a last resort,"[66] presents a somewhat different view of the role and serves to highlight the question at issue. Does advocacy offer a consistent distinction from ombudsmanship, and if so, in what way?

Gilbert and Specht note that "those who have written about the subject have actually discussed a wide range of behaviors that although referred to as advocacy, are considerably different." For example, Berger sees the term referring both to rhetoric and to orchestrated actions that are designed to alter balances of power for the benefit of a particular group. Annas and Healey compare the classical sense of advocate, which means "to summon to one's assistance, to defend, to call to one's aid," with its recently acquired connotations" of adversariness, of contentiousness, and of deliberate antagonism." Wolfensberger et al., confirm that "the advocate is generally an adversary who operates outside of the bureaucracy."[67] Thus the advocate role, similar to that of the ombudsman, is a concept that allows for numerous interpretations of its meaning, and for diversity in its application. A comparison of ombuds-manship and advocacy, therefore, cannot be made on the basis of definitions alone.

Nevertheless, a review of the literature paints some general parameters acording to which the respective roles inherent in each of the concepts may be contrasted. Annas and Healey suggest that in relation to patients' rights, "the advocate could, for example, function instead as an ombudsman." Annas and Healey appear to represent the minority interpretation, how-ever. Payne clarifies that if the ombudsman "is an advocate at all, it is only for the concept of fairness in public programs"; his goal is not to defend the individual per se. Moore goes one step further, proclaiming unequivocably: "An ombudsman is not an advocate, insofar as advocacy is incompatible with im-partiality and entails taking sides in an adversary proceeding." Mallory concurs, noting that "the ombudsman must con-sciously take a non-adversarial stance."[68]

Broderick, in support of the line of thought developed here, maintains that institutional resistance to the implementation of the ombudsman office stems from their "bad experience with adversarial advocates and the assumption that an ombudsman will inevitably be a lawyer." Regan's comparison of the pa-tients' advocate and the nursing home ombudsman further underlines the differences. He notes that while the initial methods of dispute settlement utilized by the two are quite similar, the advocate could move on to litigation which "would become fully adversarial in nature, pointing out the major dif-ferences in power and technique between the patient advocate and the ombudsman."[69]

Perhaps the most systematic comparative analysis of om-budsmanship versus advocacy is found in Verkuil's "The Om-budsman and the Limits of the Adversary System." The au-thor explains that "the ombudsman and adversary systems are substantially competing procedures for the regularization of informal processes; each is based on a different conception of the dispute resolution process and reflects different underly-ing social and political values." Furthermore, in his opinion, the predominant contemporary view that due process must resort to adversary procedures has thwarted the development of the ombudsman alternative. The strategic implications of the underlying differences are clear. "The ombudsman reconciles, reinforces and legitimates community or central decision making; the adversary system polarizes issues and fosters individualism and passive decision making."[70] Verkuil thus draws the lines, philosophically and operationally, between the two roles and their functions.

A final word needs to be mentioned as to how the literature views the relative effectiveness of the two systems. As alluded to earlier in the discussion of prison ombudsmen, the ombudsman function may tend to favor the status quo, even if it is dysfunctional to the complainant. This is the view of Theodore Lowi, according to Broderick who observed that the former perceives the ombudsman to be tied to maintenance of simple equity within the present 'disorder.' "[71]

Annas and Healey admit that while the ombudsman approach would eliminate the obstacles created by an adversary system, "the danger is that such a person would have no influence upon important decisions."[72] Moore adds that the ombudsman's "impartiality is advantageous when you need cordial access to presumptively well-intentioned administrative officials, but crippling when you need an advocate." On the other hand, he reminds us that the "techniques of advocacy may contribute unnecessarily to antagonism."

Mallory also remarked that the advocate may in certain circumstances be less effective than the ombudsman, as the former "has been hampered by lack of access to information and personnel within the bureaucratic structures." Sosin points out that successful litigative and legislative advocacy for system change may still get derailed at the point of implementation, raising the thought that the consensus approach of local ombudsmen may be required after all to overcome the informal barriers to implementation that can subvert original change goals.[73] In summation, there are clearly varying conditions under which each of the mediatory systems may prove to be more efficacious.

What Does the Nursing Home Need: Ombudsmen or Advocates?

Regan spells out the conditions under which the ombudsman or the advocate is the preferable agent for protecting patients' rights in nursing homes. He finds that the centralized complaint handling of the ombudsman avoids the case-to-case use of the courts that characterizes the adversarial approach to resolve individual grievances. As such, the ombudsman is more capable of analyzing the system as a whole and avoids introducing partisanship into nursing home relations, which "ideally should be based on confidence and trust, not hostility."[74]

At the same time, Regan warns that the profit motive of the proprietary nursing home owner is not likely to be amenable to persuasion by an ombudsman. In such a case, the patients' advocate may prove to be the preferable grievance mechanism. In conclusion, Regan declares that "the combination of the impartial ombudsman backed by the patient advocate offers the best complement to the present system of exclusive public control over the machinery for enforcing nursing home standards of care."[75]

Conclusion

The position of ombudsman has evolved from that of a state-level impartial mediator attached to a legislative body, to citizen volunteers who intervene on behalf of needy individuals. Along this evolutionary path can be seen executive ombudsmen who expedite state and local government, corrections ombudsmen who mediate in the prison system, and a plethora of other variations as disparate as welfare ombudsman, agency ombudsman, and even the public library as ombudsman. Among the new formulations of the ombudsman function is included the long-term care ombudsman for the frail elderly.

Examination of the ombudsman's development shows that the function has variously encompassed two theoretically divergent strategies: impartial mediation toward consensus and adversarial advocacy. In addition, secondary roles of helper and therapist have been incorporated within the ombudsman's role repertoire as well. It is clear that the ombudsman function portends a multiplicity of meanings, giving rise to the opportunity for the role's creative growth or ultimate confusion.

The nursing home ombudsman program draws upon disparate, and sometimes diverging, roots. The evolution of the ombudsman concept has provided a not very consistent range of roles and functions, some of which are being adopted in the field of long-term care. Just which aspects of the ombudsman idea have been incorporated into the nursing home ombudman program, and how well they work, is the subject of the research that unfolds in the remaining chapters of this book.

CHAPTER TWO

Structuring Quality Assurance Mechanisms for the Elderly in Long-Term Care

Can society guarantee the quality of care of the nation's most frail elderly—the aged residents of long-stay institutions? The task is a doubly difficult one. Not only is there little agreement about how best to assure quality care in nursing homes, but there are no commonly accepted definitions or criteria that determine what constitutes the components of acceptable care. Indeed, "it is now almost axiomatic that any thoughtful discussion of quality assurance will question what constitutes quality and how it should be defined."[1]

Beyond initial definitional disparities, the quality assurance literature reveals another barrier to the rational consideration of efforts to assure quality care. Varying methods utilized to measure "quality" may yield a range of results that vary according to the method by which they were measured. Such differences may well stem from differential foci of measurement: process or outcome.[2] They also raise serious questions of reliability and validity which further undermine the clarity of, and potential consensus on, quality care.

Still another barrier to conceptual clarity of quality assurance lies in the assessment mechanisms employed to evaluate the programs' effects. The plethora of interventive approaches from which quality assurance programmers may choose necessarily portends a wide range of possible evaluation outcomes.[3] Furthermore, a review of studies indicates that regardless of the strategy utilized, evaluation and survey methods in the field of service accountability may do little, actually, to guarantee the acceptability of long-term institutionalization.[4]

Findings from a series of studies underscore the complexity of the quality-care construct and the difficulties inherent in its operationalization.[5] At the same time, however, the limited state of knowledge in defining, measuring, and improving care in the long-term sector all necessarily point to the long-stay facility as the very arena where assurance mechanisms may be most needed.

A range of program strategies has developed to deal with such uncertainty, and to mitigate the problem of quality assurance. The following pages discuss the major models for the assurance of quality care currently in use.

The conceptual bases and major emphases of each of the assurance mechanisms are explored. The limits and potentials of their application to the health field are considered in general, as is the more specific question of their efficacy for monitoring quality in the provision of long-term care for the frail elderly. Several of them bear similar traits and may overlap in selected aspects of their strategic rationale. Indeed, the nursing home ombudsman program may be said to reflect elements of each of the quality assurance models in one way or another. The most traditional of the quality assurance mechanisms is the impartial mediation approach of the classical ombudsman.

Impartial Mediation: the Classical Ombudsman

The evolution of the concept and application of the ombudsman has been extensively reviewed in chapter 1. A brief recapitulation of the nature of ombudsmanship will serve as the basis for further discussion. It requires noting certain main points. The ombudsman originated as an independent, impartial officer of the national legislature to deal with citizens' complaints against public administration. The power of the office, however, has traditionally been to investigate and to recommend, but not to revise or reverse administrative action.

Subsequent application of the ombudsman idea has witnessed the expansion of the office into realms that were not originally considered its domain, prompting a tripartite categorization: classical, executive, and hybrid ombudsmen. The classical ombudsman constitutes the original conception of the role while the executive version refers to a political appointee who expedites administrative action in a given jurisdiction. The hybrid type, on the other hand, sees the ombudsman model extended to more specific areas, such as corrections, education, health and welfare delivery systems, and to a diversity of tasks and roles.

The classical ombudsman is most noted for adhering to an impartial mediation approach. The attainment of nonpartisan status, necessary for truly impartial mediation, is related to the degree of independence granted the office, a factor identified as the key to the ombudsman's success.

The structuring of such independence, however, may come at the expense of broad accessibility, another critical measure of ombudsman effectiveness. The problem of inaccessibility of the British Parliamentary Commissioner for Administration was noted in the previous chapter, for example. The French *mediateur,* termed by a critic as the "shackled ombudsman," is another case in point.[6] Difficulties in ensuring the mutual presence of independence and accessibility, two central characteristics necessary for the success of the impartial mediation approach, may result in potential structural strain on this quality-assurance model.

Other tensions are inherent in the classical ombudsman's operational focus as well. Hill notes that "the ombudsman was established not to alter the value system but to supplement the already existing value-maintaining agents."[7] Thus, "a normative consensus among officials, legislators and the public on standards of fair and efficient administration"[8] is a minimal condition for the functioning of this quality-assurance model. As noted, however, there may be little consensus in certain administrative domains as to acceptable standards of practice. Furthermore, as radical critics contend, such impartial mediation may simply be a means "designed to legitimate and make more palatable the existing order."[9]

An alternate role in which the classical ombudsman may realize greater success is that of a "helper to clients seeking service,"[10] rather than as a mediator of administrative abuse. Hill found in New Zealand, for example, that the handling of offensive complaints, those against service withheld by client-serving agencies, was far more common than the handling of defensive complaints, those against the abuses of maladministration. The conceptualization of the classical ombudsman as "a new kind of helping profession" not only strays from the model's original foundations, but also raises "the danger of overemphasizing the easily documented help to individuals and ignoring the long term goals of improving the system."[11] Despite a potential for a "multirole capacity,"[12] the unique contribution of the classical ombudsman is perhaps most evident in its adherence to the singular independent status of impartial mediator.

Additional dilution of this quality assurance model's potential lies in the efforts to moderate the volume of complaints handled by the ombudsman. The British and French ombudsmen cited earlier, to whom complaints must be forwarded through ministers of Parliament, are noted for their inaccessibility. The New Zealand system, on the other hand, requires the payment of a small fee with every complaint submission. This arrangement effectively discourages the poorer sections of society, and particularly the aged, from complaining "because any fee is prohibitive."[13]

Ombudsmen in numerous countries have been utilized most often by those of higher educational and occupational status, leading students of this quality-assurance model to note that ombudsmen fail to reach the persons who may be most in need of their services,[14] and "those who might need the ombudsman most are least likely to know of him and are, therefore, least likely to use his services." [15]

Given these constraints, how efficacious is the application of the classical ombudsman model to the health sector in general, and to the long-term care setting in particular? The health care sector is characterized by restraining factors that at first glance make application of an effective ombudsman questionable. Reviewing past efforts, Anderson notes "what is striking about the health-related activities of Ombuds is how little they have done." Indeed, "attempting to restructure the medical industry is a . . . formidable task and not one in which Ombudspeople have been notably successful." [16]

Foremost among the restraining factors, according to Anderson, is the primacy of the private sector in this country's health care delivery system. As mentioned earlier, the classical ombudsman's strengths lie in reviewing governmental administration and in enhancing the public channels of redress. When dealing with market-oriented mechanisms, on the other hand, the classical ombudsman model is believed to be considerably less effectual.

Second is the question of specialized professional judgment. The topic will be elaborated upon later in a discussion of consumerism as a model for quality assurance. It is significant to note here, nevertheless, that the ombudsman would have difficulty dealing with areas of professional discretion specific to the medical field. As noted in Chapter 1, the New Zealand ombudsman warned that "he must avoid straying into the area which properly belongs to the medical expert." [17]

Third are the "irremediable" aspects of life in health care institutions. The boredom, loneliness, and anxiety which may accompany the treatment period, while very real and painful to the patient, are situated outside the purview of "ombud" expertise. [18] Thus the health sector presents a number of obstacles to the successful translation of the classical ombudsman role to matters of health care.

That is not to say that there is no role for an ombudsman in health care. Anderson notes that "the medical Ombud . . .

often designated as 'patients' advocate' would probably not face basic organizational issues, but could direct his/her attention to specific complaints . . . about food, cleanliness, promptness, politeness, visiting hours, amount and manner of payment, etc. . . . and to the improvement of internal grievance machinery."[19]

Three areas that are nevertheless appropriate for ombudsman intervention at the structural level, all of which are concerned with reform of the health sector, are: establishment of standards of performance, requirement of licensing, and primary control of inspection. Such advice is tempered, however, by the observation that "as the need for such reform is greater, his ability to resolve individual grievances is less."[20]

Finally, the question of the organizational location of the medical ombud requires consideration. The British system maintains a separate post of health services ombudsman, although it has recently been held simultaneously by the national ombudsman, the Parliamentary Commissioner for Administration.[21] Anderson prefers, on the other hand, to see health-related ombudsman activities within an office of general jurisdiction. Regardless of organizational auspice, however, he maintains that "the crucial choice is not in the location of the office but in providing for sufficient qualified staff."[22]

How would a classical ombudsman fare in the complex environment of the long-term care facility? Anderson finds this quality-assurance model more appropriate to the long-stay institution than to health care per se, since the former is less dominated by doctors. He believes, on the contrary, that nurses, orderlies, and administrators are more accustomed to a chain of command and "might even welcome an Ombud." The elementary preconditions for the functioning of a long-term care ombud, furthermore, are already in place as a result of state statutes: (1) standards for nursing homes; (2) licensing; and (3) inspection requirements. It becomes clear that:

> To the extent that standards are high, inspections frequent and probing, with penalties proportionate to infractions (so that they have cred-

ibility), an Ombud would have no difficulty handling complaints against marginal defects. To the extent that the converse is true, the Ombud would have to begin his/her work by lobbying for standards, licensing, inspections, and proportionate sanctions as well as for adequate primary appeal mechanisms.[23]

The Danish ombudsman, on the other hand, reaches the opposite conclusion: "The institution of Ombudsman in its present form cannot function as a nursing home ombudsman."[24] The necessary preconditions for the effective functioning of an ombudsman in long-term care, but not yet established in Denmark, are:

1. Simplification of the administration of supervision
2. Spelling out division of responsibility (what the ombudsman can deal with)
3. Establishment of forms of cooperation for the various pertinent authorities
4. Specification of the extent of the right to appeal.

The question of the applicability of this quality-assurance model to long-term care, therefore, has not yet been decisively resolved since it varies according to contextual and content-related criteria. To what degree has the federally mandated nursing home ombudsman program in the United States approximated the classical ombudsman model's impartial mediatory focus? Anderson is of the opinion that:

Federally supported Nursing Home Ombudsman programs in a number of states have not been directed primarily to the Ombud function but have trained unpaid volunteers to visit nursing homes. In addition to primary functions of providing companionship, information, and advocacy, it is hoped that the volunteers may be able to identify and forward complaints. The salaried head of a given Nursing Home Ombudsman program, however, has no independent capacity for investigation and so the complaints are usually referred to the standard governmental licensing and regulatory bodies. Consequently, the Nursing Home Ombud programs do not serve as an Ombudsmanic fail-safe mechanism to protect against the breakdown of the standard control devices.[25]

How, then, would the ombudsman model be most fruitfully translated to the field of long-term care? Anderson requires that all ombudsmen, including those placed in long-term care, adhere to the classical origins of this quality-assurance model as much as possible. It is his position that:

> Careful precautions should be taken to maintain the purity of the con-
> cept—not as an idle formalism, but because it is the peculiar combina-
> tion of characteristics of an Ombud which permit him to perform his
> special function of using the feedback from complaints to correct defi-
> ciencies in the other control mechanisms of government.[26]

The limits and apparent complexity of the ombudsman model have led some advocates of quality long-term care to turn to the government in quest of quality assurance.

Governmental Regulation and Patients' Rights

"As an old person enters a nursing home, very often the concept of rights is packed up and sent away along with all other life-long valuables."[27] To prevent just such phenomena, advocates for nursing home residents have increasingly looked to the federal government to issue regulations that recognize, enforce, and protect their basic rights to quality of care, dignity, and quality of life. Even so, the role and utility of governmental regulation and statutory empowerment as a quality-assurance model have been subject to a variety of criticisms.

Wilson, for example, recognizes the ubiquity of deprivation of personal rights and liberties of nursing home patients but questions whether such rights are enforceable. First, federally regulated patient rights may be waived when medically contraindicated. This provision permits negligent facilities a potential escape clause from obedience to federal law. Secondly, the less tangible rights of exercising citizenship, recommending changes, being treated with dignity and individuality, and so on, are very difficult to enforce through the regular inspection process. Finally, and most significantly,

The elderly nursing home patient whose rights have been aggrieved is prevented from bringing suit by his isolation from the community, including lawyers; his lack of physical energy and psychic combativeness; the problems of proof where staff will unite against aged and drugged complainants; the law of damages which places small value on injury to those whose actuarial life expectancies are zero; and his probable lack of money to pay for legal representation.[28]

These very real obstacles lead Wilson to conclude: "If the patients' bill of rights concept is to mean more to the elderly than a show of good intentions, it is vital that some means of enforcement which is accessible to patients be established." In their review of the Illinois Nursing Home Reform Act of 1979, Daley and Jost similarly cite the potential of regulated residents' rights, but nevertheless conclude the law is worthless without concomitant commitment from enforcing agencies, relatives, and friends of nursing home patients.[29]

Caldwell and Kapp, on the other hand, question the inadvertent harm which protective regulation may create. "Regulation may perpetuate unreasonable burdens, such as paper trail documentation, or result in counterproductive limitations which violate rights in unintended ways."[30] As an example they cite the defensive medicine which many physicians practice as protection against malpractice suits. "The consequent restriction on residents' freedom may ultimately exceed any protection which the proposed 'right' could have assured." Thus,

Regulations may or may not be a source of rights. They do, however, offer important protections. The legal protections that proposed regulations seek to secure for patients are necessary to prevent abuses of power. The incontrovertible fact, however, is that the most comprehensively written and vigorously enforced regulations in the world can only work to a small degree to protect dependents from abuses.[31]

Lastly, in a review of the federal regulations governing the physician who practices in the long-term care facility, Loeser et al. conclude that statutory promulgations have little to do with the quality of care.[32] Instead, such regulations breed time-consuming paper work, which reduces patient contact hours.

It can be seen, therefore, that there is considerable literature which reflects ambivalently on the efficacy of federal regulation and statutory empowerment as a quality assurance model. Nevertheless, the trend has been toward more, rather than less, regulation of nursing-home-related matters.

Statutory empowerment of those who protect the rights of nursing home residents has evolved over the last decade, starting from broad federal legislation and extending to subsequent state statutes for specific matters of long-term care. As reviewed by the National Citizens' Coalition for Nursing Home Reform:

> The first federal bill of rights in the mid 1970's largely expressed First Amendment rights and liberties, addressing such concerns as the right to meet with people, to exercise rights of citizenship, to enjoy religious liberty, and to receive and send mail unopened. More recent state laws have expanded the protected rights to include financial issues and the right to receive health care in a facility meeting federal and state standards. Recent state laws have also recognized the need for strong and varied mechanisms to enforce protected rights.[33]

Federal legislative foundations upon which residents' rights suits may be based include cases of (1) discrimination based on race, color, or national original (prohibited by Title VI of the Civil Rights Act of 1964); and (2) discrimination based on handicap (prohibited by s. 504 of the Rehabilitation Act of 1973).

The National Citizens' Coalition for Nursing Home Reform also documented a wide range of legislated and proposed state statutes currently aimed at augmenting the more general federal regulation of nursing home residents' rights. A selected review of such state legislation revealed that various attempts are being made to empower statutorily the regulation of access to facilities and patient records, adult protection and abuse reporting, alternatives to institutions, complaint and abuse reporting procedure, cost containment, fines, guardianship, inspection, insurance, licensure, varying aspects of Medicaid financing, medication, ombudsman functions, receivership, reimbursement, residents' councils, residents' rights, and transfer of nursing home patients.

In light of the limitations of impartial mediation, the alternative of statutory empowerment of regulating agents seems to have become a preferred method for long-term care quality assurance. Governmental regulation may fall short, however, at a critical point in the assurance process. Sosin points out that legislation and court mandates are necessary but not necessarily sufficient criteria for implementing quality assurance. Experience shows that desired changes may be compromised by local resistance.[34] Sosin suggests, therefore, that legal mandates need to be followed by a range of advocacy roles and activities if indeed they are to be implemented. Discussion of such "implementation advocacy" leads to the consideration of voluntarism and consumerism as models for quality assurance.

Voluntarism

One of the primary ways proposed to enhance the intent of statutorily regulated patients' rights is through the application of volunteer-based strategies. A selected sample of sources indicates that voluntarism offers significant potential benefits to the task of quality assurance. The adoption of such voluntary advocacy activity, on the other hand, must be carried out with awareness of some strategic dilemmas that may result in divergence from initial action goals.

Etzioni sees voluntarism, which he terms the "third sector," as a major alternative to current institutional arrangements for the implementation of policy:

Greater reliance on the third sector, both as a way of reducing government on all levels and as a way of involving the private sector in the service of domestic missions, would be significantly more effective than either expanding the federal or other levels of government or dropping them on the private sector.[35]

Berger and Neuhaus similarly recognize the role of voluntary associations as mediating institutions, citing "wherever possible, public policy should utilize mediating structures for the realization of social purposes."[36] As a complement to their call, Langton confirms that with increased importance placed on such mediating institutions there has been a dramatic growth in the number of citizen advocacy movements since the 1960s.[37]

Alongside such support for voluntary advocacy, however, are varied warnings as to the misapplication or misuse of voluntarism. Jordan has complained that "voluntarism has been caught in the straitjacket of service. It has become fixated on the concept of service provision to the neglect of advocacy that deals with the root causes that create the demand for service."[38] O'Connell similarly notes:

> There are multiple roles the voluntary sector plays, but anything which compromises or detracts from efforts to influence public policy diminishes the sector's capacity to function in the role society most depends on it to perform.[39]

Adams, on the other hand, warns of "the evil of making too great claims for the competency of voluntary association," maintaining instead that the voluntaristic principle is primarily for "prophetic purposes."[40]

How may the contradictions mentioned here be resolved so as to promote efficient voluntary advocacy as a model for quality assurance? Langton suggests that it is first efficacious to distinguish between the two dominant types of advocacy that volunteers are enlisted to enact.[41] The first is subjective advocacy which has "a direct and relatively exclusive benefit to the advocating institution." The second is prophetic advocacy and refers to "proposals concerned with correcting unjust conditions in society and which will have little or no direct benefit to the institution." Thus, in regard to quality assurance, the voluntaristic model need first clarify which type and what degree of advocacy it can realistically be expected to pursue.

In addition, Langton notes that the fruitful application of voluntarism requires "a healthy balance between advocacy and service functions."[42] The question remains, however, whether such balance may indeed be attained, or whether advocacy must come at the expense of service, and vice versa.

Vosburgh relates these concerns to the deinstitutionalization phenomenon. He sees a place for watchdog functions (which may address aspects of both subjective and prophetic advocacy) and for service functions, which in this case may be termed a kind of individual or case advocacy. In discussing the latter among deinstitutionalized mental patients, he notes that a volunteer advocate can play a positive role by "indicating to the professional what things about the course of diagnosis and treatment the client has found to be unclear or has developed doubts about."[43] However, "in order to qualify for this type of advocacy, a volunteer would have to achieve a detailed knowledge of procedures, rules and regulations governing the service activity."[44]

The strategic dilemmas to which a voluntary quality assurance model may fall prey have also been noted.[45] First, to what extent can a volunteer be expected to press the interests of a patient/resident against opposition in a facility which sponsors his activity? Indeed, is the work of volunteer advocates most useful if they are part of the agency monitored, or if they are external to it?

Second, how may the volunteer handle the questioning of professional judgment and experience, particularly on the basis of a patient's complaint which may be lacking a full understanding of what has been done on his behalf? This dilemma further implies that decisions must be made about the efficacy of ongoing adversariness by the volunteer advocate for the assurance of responsiveness to clients.

Finally, does advocacy for individuals result unintentionally in the phenomenon of "queue-jumping," in which some clients achieve greater response at the expense of others? Such advocacy on behalf of individuals may come at the expense of advocacy for general systemic reform, and may inadvertently perpetuate some root causes of the delivery system's dysfunction. Two positive points need to be raised, however, before concluding the discussion of voluntarism as a model for quality assurance. Vosburgh and Hyman confirm that volunteers are among the very few who are in a position to view the patients' experience in the totality and thus offer a unique perspective from which to advocate for them. Furthermore, violations of dignity, which are not systematically addressed in human service agencies, are among the easiest difficulties for other lay persons to discover.[46] Thus, the volunteer provides useful functions that enhance the task of quality assurance.

The application of voluntarism as a model for quality assurance entails strategic dilemmas at the level of policy-making alongside selected advantages in the realm of personal advocacy. Critics of voluntarism have cited the lack of power available to the volunteer advocate as a source of this quality-assurance model's lack of impact. The next model, consumerism as a form of quality assurance, is concerned with the very area where voluntarism hesitates to tread: the building of constituencies, coalitions, and organized advocacy movements.

Consumerism

Consumerism, or the organized demand for accountability and consumer quality assessment, is a field that has seen great growth in recent decades.[47] The approach of citizens' involvement in decisions that affect them has spread across all major institutions in this society, including the field of health. As Huttmann summarizes, "it has been recognized that the public demands the right to participate in the decisions affecting health care."[48]

The translation of consumerism to the health field in general, and to the long-term care facility in particular, has been difficult because of the long-standing tradition of physicians' authority, or the legitimated right to direct interaction with patients.[49] Parsons underscores that there exists a competence gap between physician and patient that creates an inherently asymmetrical authority relation between the two as regards knowledge of specific health care functions.[50]

Freidson, however, indicates that there are other explanations for the establishment of physicians' authority. He writes that such authority does not derive solely from expertise, as Parsons suggests, but rather from the institutionalization of that expertise "into something similar to bureaucratic office." The medical profession's organized autonomy and its dominance over the division of labor in health exert "a special and biased influence on the planning and financing of the services of the general field within which it is located."[51]

Freidson's analysis suggests that the successful application of consumerism as a model for quality assurance will require more than consumer interest or concern. Rather, the use of organizing and power-related tactics is indicated if a consumer approach is to make an impact upon such a powerfully entrenched professional discipline as medicine. Physicians' control over all decisions affecting patients may well yield only to equally organized constituencies and effectively orchestrated uses of power. The strategic implication of this arrangement is to create a social movement out of the many but disparate consumer and citizen groups expressing common concerns.

Predicated upon such assumptions, the National Citizens' Coalition for Nursing Home Reform has attempted to apply a consumer movement approach to the field of long-term care. Numerous publications by this organization provide technical and ideational assistance in the effort to attain a powerful constituency among consumers of extended care facilities and their advocates.[52]

On the local level the consumer approach has been fully integrated into at least one of the state nursing home ombudsman programs, and partially adopted in others. Citizens for Better Care, a nursing home consumer and advocacy organization in Michigan, operates a federally mandated long-term care ombudsman program.[53] Other state nursing home ombudsman programs, such as those in Oregon and Minnesota, maintain extensive ties with citizens' consumer organizations, but are not formally contracted to them. At the same time, still other states have nursing home consumer organizations, such as Citizens for Better Care, of Illinois, and Iowans for Better Care, that are unrelated to the states' formal long-term care ombudsman program.

How ripe is the field of long-term care for a consumer social movement approach? Documented difficulties cast a questionable light upon the successful application of a consumer movement among the aged for better health care. Haug notes:

> In a period when the public is increasingly challenging traditional relations with professionals, questioning the authority of physicians and taking a consumerist stance in encounters with medical care providers . . . research indicates that those aged 60 and above are more likely to adhere to an acceptance of such authority, both in attitude and behavior.[54]

There are indications of change, however, "because future cohorts of the elderly are likely to be better educated and thus more medically knowledgeable," and more apt to "carry over tendencies rejecting authority."[55] Neugarten also maintains that the aged of the future will be more active and have higher expectations concerning community participation and the satisfaction of their needs.[56]

The consumerist approach to quality assurance of long-term care may thus be currently tempered by the hesitance of the aged to advocate against doctors' orders, and by the very inability of the frail institutionalized elderly to act on their own behalf as active consumer representatives. The alternative to this current shortcoming, the use of consumer advocates in place of, or in additon to, long-term care consumers themselves, overlaps in principle with the use of delegated authority by means of boards of visitors.

Delegated Authority: Boards of Visitors

There is a relative paucity of literature on the use of delegated authority in the form of boards of visitors to provide quality assurance. Two examples of this model in practice are boards of visitors for the mentally disabled in state institutions in New York and the board of visitors in Great Britain's prison system. Both provide interesting analogous experience to nursing home ombudsman programs.

Unlike the classical ombudsman model, boards of visitors put the mediation process into operation through active visitation at the facility level by volunteers with authority delegated by the government. Unlike the consumer movement model, these visitor-advocates, who may include families and friends of mental patients, as well as former patients (but no former offenders in the British case), strive more for impartiality than for adversarial advocacy. The result is a combination of elements common to each of the quality-assurance models discussed above—the ombudsman concept combined with voluntarism and some consumerist principles, backed up by governmental regulation. The following paragraphs explore the means which enable the boards of visitors to function, and whether they indeed provide quality assurance.

In New York State, the board of visitors is an independent, seven-member, unsalaried citizen body that is appointed to each of the state's mental hygiene facilities. "Conceptually, this lay body remains the conscience of the community within the mental institution."[57] As noted by the chairman of the New York State Commission on Quality Care for the Mentally Disabled, however, these fifty-six boards of lay persons charged with performing complex functions (including investigation of charges against facility directors and allegations of patient abuse) "were thrown into an extremely complicated human services delivery system with no orientation, training or education in the tasks they were charged by law with performing."[58]

While the boards of visitors are appointed by the governor

and have statutory authority to perform their function, questions have been raised as to their ability to perform within the confines of a lack of extrastatutory support. Sections 7.33 and 13.33 of the Mental Hygiene Law indeed conferred upon the boards the requirement to conduct periodic unannounced visits and

1. The power to investigate all charges against the director and all cases of alleged patient abuse or mistreatment made against any employee.
2. The power to interview patients and employees of the facility in pursuit of such investigations.
3. The power, in accordance with civil practice law rules, to subpoena witnesses under oath, and require the production of any books or papers deemed relevant to the investigation.[59]

However, reality revealed a different set of outcomes to the efforts of the boards of visitors:

> Requests for legal assistance in subpoenaing witnesses and taking testimony under oath, which Boards are authorized to do under law, were frequently denied because ready resources with which to respond were unavailable. The large volume of reports compiled by the Boards on conditions within the facilities were scarcely acknowledged and even more rarely read. Thus, critical insights of dedicated volunteers had little impact on improving the quality of care.[60]

The "obvious limitations of an all-volunteer system for performing comprehensive monitoring and advocacy" led the governor to enact additional means to assure quality of care, and not to rely upon the boards of visitors alone. Thus a state-level Board of Visitors Advisory Council, a Mental Hygiene Medical Review Board, and a Commission on Quality of Care for the Mentally Disabled, composed of three full-time commissioners, were created to augment the well-intentioned but overtaxed system of boards of visitors at the facility level.

The English boards of visitors for that nation's penal system reveal similar tendencies. There are currently 110 different boards composed of about a dozen persons each, appointed by the Home Secretary, whose office oversees the country's Prison Department. The boards' duties include general inspection of the prison facilities and regime to "satisfy themselves as to the state of the prison premises, the administration of the prison and the treatment of the prisoners."[61] Boards of visitors are expected to visit the prison frequently, are given access to all facilities, personnel, and records, and may visit at any time of day or night with no advance notice.

In fulfilling their function as boards of visitors, "members must be careful to avoid becoming identified as either prisoners' or the prison staff's public advocates." Nevertheless, and in spite of the structured attempt to overcome this problem, there is still "major controversy about . . . whether they are sufficiently independent to perform their many functions." In sum,

> It is difficult to reach a conclusion about the impact of Boards of Visitors. Some Boards work quite hard and can be so assertive that they are resented by the prison administration. Other Boards do little more than make cursory inspections. In neither case can the Board order sweeping changes in prison policy or facilities. But this does not mean that Boards serve no useful function. If nothing else they remove some of the secrecy and isolation that seems to flourish in many penal institutions. By giving responsible community members access to a prison and its inhabitants, Boards of Visitors can help demystify what goes on inside the walls.[62]

In the nursing home home ombudsman program in the United States, two states, Florida and North Carolina, have modeled their long-term care quality-assurance programs after the delegated authority model. Indeed, the Florida Long Term Care Ombudsman Committee framework, which is most similar to the boards of visitors concept, is often cited as one of this country's most effective nursing home ombudsman programs.[63] Nevertheless, a program model which structures quality assurance through delegated statutory authority has not, in the main, become the prototype of state nursing home ombudsman programs.

A quality-assurance model that operates outside the mandated state nursing home ombudsman structure is the last model to be considered: participatory democracy through resident and family councils.

Participatory Democracy: Resident and Family Councils

Participatory democracy implies the taking part by citizens in making and shaping decisions that affect them in their day-to-day lives. As a political theory it dates back to Rousseau's *Social Contract*. More recently it has seen renewed interest in the form of worker self-management, student participation in higher educational policy, and "maximum feasible participation" of the war on poverty era. The fostering of democratization of decision-making has been linked both to education for self-determination and to maximization of individual political efficacy.[64]

The renewed interest in the values of participatory democracy has not been totally absent from the field of long-term care, where it is argued that "residents can and should share in making the decisions that affect their lives and govern their destiny."[65] The mechanism that has become associated with participatory democracy within the long-stay institution is the residents' council. Silverstone defines the purpose of the residents' council thus:

> To serve as a vehicle for residents to exercise their rights and protect their interests by participating fully in the decisions and tasks which affect their everyday lives, both in the home and the outside community.[66]

The residents' council model has not achieved universal support among nursing home administrators, however. Shore admits that:

> While we know the value of resident participation in activity programs, we do not always feel secure in enabling our residents to actually have a means for group decision-making and self-government.[67]

Furthermore, even where they have been enacted, "the councils have all too often been perfunctory, exist in name only or are the front, or rubber stamp, for the administrator."[68]

Councils have also been criticized as unrealistic in light of the residents' frail condition. Silverstone refutes this contention, however, claiming that residents' councils are capable of involving all residents regardless of infirmity if democratically organized.[69] A more practical shortcoming in the council as a participatory mechanism in the nursing home is that residents may have a fear of reprisal should they participate.[70] The residents' council is thus not entirely free of limitations.

To what degree can the residents' council serve as a model for quality assurance? Newmark views the council as a potential means for quality assurance as well as an interpersonal human relations medium. He states the functions of the council thus:

1. To serve as a means of bringing problems and grievances to the director's attention.
2. To help plan the leisure time program.
3. To make suggestions regarding other activities in the home.[71]

In summarizing the role the council actually played, however, Newmark cities mostly developmental and process oriented benefits over the benefits related to quality assurance:

1. The council brought the residents together in an organized way.
2. It gave them a feeling of their importance to other people in the home.
3. It provided an opportunity to share ideas and experiences, to talk things over, for the improvement of the home.
4. It served as a channel for complaints and grievances.
5. It was a learning experience.
6. Through the council the residents got a feeling of belonging.
7. It offered them a chance to help plan programs.[72]

Shore, too, presents evidence that the residents' council serves as a therapeutic tool, as opposed to a quality assurance model. He cites the experience of one elderly resident with a resident council as follows:

> Members of the resident council welcome new residents. We try to give them the feeling of belonging, of being among friends. The resident council helps plan leisure time programs; religious guidance plays a large part in the life of the home. We meet regularly with our director. We discuss food problems, recreational programs, activities for busy, skillful hands are encouraged.[73]

A recent publication by Parker and Shields, on the other hand, stresses the quality-assurance role of this form of participatory democracy in the nursing home:

> The basic premise of the Council is that residents should share in planning and controlling their lives. . . . The Resident Council acts as a social stethoscope of the home, reflecting the priority concerns of the resident community, arrived at as democratically as possible. A Resident Council can seek changes in living conditions for the residents, prevent services from deteriorating, act as an educational tool, convey the needs and preferences of the residents and represent residents to the outside community. In addition, residents can become informed and educated about facility policies, community resources, and the rules and regulations of the long term care system by using the Council as a forum for guest speakers.[74]

A variation on the resident council model is the family advisory council[75] or organizations of friends and relatives.[76] Such bodies range from consensual, in-house organs to bona fide consumer movements like the Virginia Friends and Relatives of Nursing Home Residents, which identifies itself in its brochure as "an advocacy group for nursing home residents who are often isolated, powerless to change their situation and without a collective voice." As such, they variously represent aspects of the models discussed so far, and offer the same themes on quality-assurance structures that have already been considered.

The residents' council and its offshoots offer an experience in participatory democracy to the residents of the long-term care facility. The determination as to whether they can also serve as an effective means to assure the residents' quality of care, however, must await more empirically oriented research and evaluation. One such study recently completed by the American Association of Homes for the Aging probed the involvement of nursing home ombudsmen with resident governance in homes for the aging.

The study "undertook a survey of nursing home ombudsmen to assess the extent of ombudsman interest and involvement in resident council organization, activity and training."[77] It was hypothesized that ombudsman involvement in the operation of a residents' council would negatively affect the council's relationship with the facility administrator, that where there was such involvement it would be limited to individual complaints, and that such involvement was dependent upon the existence of volunteer ombudsman programs.

The major findings indicated that while most ombudsmen found involvement in residents' councils an appropriate activity for the ombudsman program, very few spent time in such involvement. In the few ombudsman projects which aided in the development of residents' councils, no negative effects concerning facility administrator relationships were reported. Furthermore, involvement did focus on individual complaint resolution, but was not discernibly dependent upon volunteer activity. It would seem from the findings of this study that while participatory democracy can be conceived as a potential quality assurance mechanism, long-term care ombudsmen have not currently incorporated it into their modus operandi.

CHAPTER THREE
Study Methodology

This study was conducted during the period November 1979 through December 1981 and encompassed a two-pronged approach. The first stage examined the experience of the New York City nursing home patient ombudsman program. The second surveyed the providers of long-term care ombudsman services and members of the long-term care service network in each of the fifty states.

The New York City ombudsman program is an Older Americans Act project funded by both the New York City Department for the Aging and the New York State Office for the Aging. The program was initiated in March of 1978 and operates under the auspice of the Community Council of Greater New York. All its ombudsmen, save for administrative and supervisory staff, serve as volunteers recruited from the local community who are independent of nursing home ties. The program's stated purposes are: (1) to make the nursing home a part of the community; (2) to provide a process by which patients' complaints can be expressed and resolved; and (3) to seek information from various sources to answer residents' questions about their care or benefits.

In broad terms, the research inquired whether the program succeeded in:

1. Improving the day-to-day life of individual residents
2. Bringing about systemic and operational changes benefiting all nursing home patients

3. Preventing the recurrence of service deficiencies
4. Providing an effective mechanism for resolving residents' grievances
5. Assisting in the protection of residents' rights
6. Establishing a community support system of interested organizations in the target communities that would ensure the continuity and viability of the public scrutiny objectives.

The second study included similar objectives on a national scale and addressed elements both external and internal to ombudsman programs. External issues encompassed demographic characteristics, legislative/regulatory incentives and disincentives, and interorganizational influences. Internal issues related to program-specific or intraorganizational factors such as the nature of auspice, problems addressed, staffing patterns, service methods, and accountability mechanisms.

The ultimate objectives of both studies were, first, simply to ascertain whether the program works or not and second, to contribute to a model of practice for community-sponsored, volunteer ombudsman programs.

From a planning and evaluative perspective, the study design had to be concerned with the following programmatic questions:

1. *Feasibility.* Is the program viable in terms of prevailing administrative practices and their concurrent political and interorganizational constraints?
2. *Accountability.* Can the program overcome systemic resistances and marshal support among its potential beneficiaries?
3. *Adequacy.* Is the program's capacity to intervene commensurate with the service problems it has to confront?
4. *Effectiveness.* Are the program's preestablished objectives attainable as a result of the program's activities?

Both studies had to follow by necessity an *ex post facto* design since no pretests were initially built into the ombudsman program. Moreover, the research project was launched well after the program was into an advanced implementation stage. The studies therefore utilized retrospective information of three types:

1. Original data obtained by means of structured survey instruments
2. Original information collected through semistructured interviews
3. Secondary information derived from unobtrusive and secondary sources.

This chapter will review in detail the methodology followed by each of the two studies.

The New York City Study

Preliminary Activity

Prior to construction of the research instruments, a series of exploratory/orientation sessions was conducted with staff of the New York City nursing home patient ombudsman program between November and January of 1979–80. These meetings allowed research staff members to make themselves known to, and become familiar with, key personnel who related directly or indirectly to the ombudsman program. During this time, the research proposal was systematically reviewed, key research questions clarified, methodological and technical details ironed out, and respondent populations and samples defined in terms of size and identity. These initial meetings also proved to be critically important in reducing much of the inevitable hesitation and stress that tend to surface when an exogenous research initiative is virtually imposed on a direct service program.

The Survey Instruments

Structured research questionnaires were directed at four potential respondent groups:

1. Program sponsors: advisory board members
2. Program actors: active volunteer ombudsmen
3. Institutional representatives: participating long-term care staff
   a) Administrators
   b) Directors of nursing
   c) Directors of social services
4. Program beneficiaries: residents/patients in long-term care facilities.

Instrument pretesting was performed at two levels: draft instruments were individually reviewed question-by-question with the ombudsman project director and one of the program supervisors. The feedback, in the form of observations and suggestions, proved very useful in altering the "semantic display" of individual questions, adding and deleting certain questions, and tightening up the "forced choice" items so as better to reflect actual program experience in New York City.

At the second, more formal level of pretesting, arrangements were worked out for research staff to pilot test the instruments at a nursing home participating in the Westchester nursing home patient ombudsman program, an area not covered by the study. This allowed the conducting of face-to-face interviews with directors of nursing and social services and actual residents, the nursing home administrators, and ombudsmen themselves. The Advisory Board (Committee of Auspice) questionnaire was pilot tested on former advisory members of the New York City ombudsman program. This level of testing enabled research staff to refine further the draft instruments in terms both of substantive content and schedule design. Furthermore, it ensured against any contagious effect spreading to the later phase of formal interviewing since all testing avoided contact with current members of the designated survey populations and samples.

The final survey schedules were a combination of closed- and open-ended items aimed at providing opportunities for the six different key study groups to describe their experiences and views in detail. They covered the following content categories:

1. Long-term care facility identifying information
2. Attitudes toward nursing home ombudsman services
3. Experiential information concerning contacts with the volunteer ombudsman
4. Evaluative assessments of program performance
5. Personal data.

Completion time ranged between twenty and seventy-five minutes.

The Semistructured Interviews

Semistructured guides were utilized for all interviews with secondary sponsors of the ombudsman program. They encompassed key members of the interorganizational support network (representatives of legal aid offices, the state health department, area/state agencies on aging, nursing home associations, local voluntary advocacy groups, and so on). The interview guide solicited information about: the nature and quality of interorganizational relationships; needed changes in these relationships; the adequacy of feedback concerning program activities; perceived strengths and weaknesses of the program; importance of program continuation; aspects of the program that needed change; appropriate roles for ombudsmen, and the importance of gaining additional program authority.

Unobtrusive Data Sources

Content analysis of secondary program data sources included review of the ombudsman contact registers, monthly summaries of ombudsman activities, minutes of ombudsman and Committee of Auspice monthly meetings, and a newsletter called *Ombudsnews*. All program materials available January 1, 1979, through March 30, 1980, were included in the analysis.

Content analysis guides were developed to measure the nature of complaints as well as the focus, level, and type of communication utilized by volunteer ombudsmen in attending to complaints by residents of nursing homes. A unit of five graduate student social workers assigned to the research project performed the actual secondary analysis based on the guides developed by research staff. A series of research training sessions and workshops incorporating elements of role-playing, trial runs, lecture format, and discussion preceded this phase of the research.

The ultimate informational value of program sources was limited due to repeated modifications in the design of the contact registers and monthly summaries that occurred during the life of the program, as well as the difficulties inherent in having volunteers implement the record-keeping. The variability in the quantity and quality of such program records reinforced the importance of original survey data serving as a major source of information for program assessment.

The Respondent Groups

The survey was directed at four study populations:

1. *Program sponsors.* These included both direct and indirect sponsors of ombudsman program activities. Direct primary sponsors were the actual salaried staff that administered, supervised, and trained the volunteer community ombudsmen as well as the advisory board members (Committee of Auspice members) representing three sections of New York City (Brooklyn, Queens, and Far Rockaway). It is noted that subsequent to the period of survey activity the committees of auspice were reduced to two in number, representing Brooklyn and Queens.

   Indirect or secondary sponsors were agency and organizational representatives not involved in the day-to-day operation of the program, which tended to lend some supportive function, including the provision of program legitimation, backing during the complaint resolution process and information on specific grievance issues that might surface. Included here were: the New York

City Department for the Aging, New York State Office for the Aging, New York State Department of Health, New York City Human Resources Administration, New York City Legal Aid Services for the Aged (Brooklyn and Queens), New York State Office of the Special Prosecutor, voluntary community advocacy groups for the aged, borough presidents' offices (Brooklyn and Queens), and associations of homes for the aged.

2. *Program actors.* These were the volunteer community ombudsmen. The study focused on those volunteers who were active at the time of questionnaire administration.

3. *Institutional representatives.* This category included three subgroups of long-term care facility staff: (a) nursing home administrators, (b) directors of nursing, and (c) directors of social services. At the time of questionnaire administration, twenty-three long-term care facilities were or recently had been participating in the nursing home patient ombudsman program in New York City. They were situated in the boroughs of Brooklyn and Queens.

4. *Program beneficiaries.* This cateogry included both users and non-users of the ombudsman program service. They were elderly patients/residents in fifteen long-term care facilities participating in the ombudsman program in Brooklyn and Queens (excluding Far Rockaway).

Because of the limited sizes of these four respondent groups (save for program beneficiaries), they were approached in their totality. Structured questionnaires were completed by 77.4 percent of active advisory board members, 88.4 percent of long-term care facility staff, and 83.3 percent of the active volunteer ombudsmen. The latter figure is an approximation due to the high turnover and unanticipated period of inactivity among volunteer participants.

Interviews with residents of long-term care facilities were conducted by means of incidental sampling procedures. This non-random approach was inevitable due to the high percentage of patients who suffer from organic brain disturbances, severe physical disabilities, and language impediments. Furthermore, confidentiality regulations required that the researchers not single out the residents registered as past users of the ombudsman program service.

The five-member interview team conducted fifteen interviews with residents in each of fourteen currently active long-term care facilities in the boroughs of Brooklyn and Queens. This approached virtual universal sampling of participating facilities at the time of questionnaire administration. Due to the possible negative consequences of sending a survey team into an unresponsive facility, interviews were not conducted in one institution that was at that time faced with probable litigation proceedings. Therefore, a completion rate of 93.3 percent was realized among the institutionalized aged sample. Patients capable of being interviewed were identified by long-term care staff or were personally approached by the interviewers. This procedure would suggest that the resultant sample is biased in the direction of the more active and alert residents.

It is worthy of note that all four study populations increased considerably from the time of writing the original proposal to the actual implementation of the research study. This was due to the rapid expansion of the New York City nursing home patient ombudsman program. As a result, the research staff determined to make every effort to alter its scope and include the increased number of participants in its research design.

Areas of Research

All activities carried out in this study were guided by five major substantive areas and their study variables that comprised the investigatory framework:

1. Program Descriptive
   a) Categories of complaints
   b) Grievance resolution rates
   c) Client satisfaction indices
2. Grievance Process
   a) Initiation of intervention
   b) Acceptance of intervention
   c) Communication with patient
   d) Investigation of complaint
   e) Determination of validity of complaint
   f) Case-finding and complaint sources

3. Program Operation
   a) Effectiveness of:
      (1) Recruitment procedures
      (2) Training sessions
      (3) Retention methods
      (4) "Recycling" of volunteers
      (5) Public education function
      (6) Information and referral function
      (7) Public policy formation function
      (8) Feedback procedures
      (9) Reporting mechanisms
   b) Adequacy of:
      (1) Funding
      (2) Volunteer/facility matching
      (3) Supervision
      (4) Back-up services
4. Interorganizational Relations
   a) Access negotiation to long-term care facilities
   b) Boundaries of intervention
   c) Linkages with licensing, regulating agencies, advocacy, client groups
   d) Strategies of community influence
   e) Decision-making processes concerning:
      (1) Goal-setting
      (2) Program definitions
      (3) Monitoring
   f) Coalition formation
   g) Determinants of intersystemic conflict
5. Role Prescription
   a) Role socialization
   b) Self-perception
   c) Effectiveness of role specializations
   d) Role acceptance and resistance
   e) Definitions of role "success"
   f) Role satisfaction
   g) Role routines
   h) Range of discretionary decision-making.

Data Collection

Advisory board members (committees of auspice) underwent a group administration of their protocol during their scheduled monthly meetings. A follow-up mail survey was then carried out for those members who had not attended the monthly meetings. Individuals who considered themselves to be active members and had attended at least one monthly meeting prior to questionnaire administration were included in this category.

Semistructured interviewing commenced December 1979 and was completed in October 1980. Structured interviewing commenced in February 1980 and was completed on July 30, 1980. Setting appointments and completing interviews met with varying degrees of resistance, fear, and apathy by long-term care staff and to a lesser degree by residents and patients.

Due to the physical and mental status of many patients, advance appointments were not made, but requests for interviews were made during field visits to each long-term care facility.

Data Analysis

Univariate and nonparametric forms of data analysis performed included the usual descriptive statistics, simple frequency distributions, cross-tabulations, simple and partial correlations, as well as one-way and two-way analysis of variance. During the course of the study new variables were generated which were logical combinations of existing ones, and ranked variables were differentially weighted to simplify and aggregate necessary information. In general, statistical procedures were utilized that facilitated arriving at intra- and intercorrelational measures for the six respondent categories.

The judgments of a ten-member expert panel were utilized to validate individual scale items for several composite measures of aspects of the ombudsman program. The expert panel was composed of faculty, researchers, and practitioners throughout New York State and Connecticut with acknowledged expertise in the field of social welfare.

The National Study

Study Design

This study of nursing home ombudsman programs across the country also followed by necessity an *ex post facto* survey design, as no appropriate base-line data or prior measures existed at the inception of the research. Data collection stemmed principally from structured questionnaires mailed to targeted respondents. Semistructured interviews conducted during observational on-site visits to nine selected state programs supplemented the questionnaire data. Additional unobtrusive data in the form of reports and other printed material solicited from the state ombudsmen further expanded the primary data derived from the questionnaire.

Two foci of inquiry were encompassed in the study design: measurement of perspectives on the current status of the nursing home ombudsman program in each state, and consideration of varying views concerning the future design of such programs. Two major groups of respondents were addressed: the state nursing home ombudsmen, and representatives of the long-term care delivery system. The composition of this latter group, the "long-term care network," as it is usually termed here, will be further enumerated. The study design thus allowed for a survey of the perceptions of principal actors in the nursing home ombudsman program, combined with supportive field observational and unobtrusive data.

The Study Sample

Preliminary activity encompassed the identification and compilation of respondent sources to comprise the sampling frame from which the study sample was subsequently selected. Initial contacts with the office of the federal ombudsman, the National Citizens' Coalition for Nursing Home Reform, the American Health Care Associaton, and the American Association of Homes for the Aging, as well as extensive searches for current data on state government functionaries, produced a comprehensive sampling frame. Study groups for this investigation were identified as follows:

Group A. State ombudsmen
Group B. Long-term care network
  1. Older Americans advocacy assistance programs (legal services)
  2. State units on aging
  3. State departments of health
  4. State departments of welfare
  5. State associations of not-for-profit long-term care facilities
  6. State associations of proprietary long-term care facilities
  7. State community action interest groups for the elderly

Contact was made with representatives of each study group in each state where the category was operative. Thus state ombudsmen, commissioners on aging, commissioners of health, and commissioners of welfare from each of the fifty states plus the District of Columbia were approached. Legal services developers were similarly approached except in Alaska, which does not sponsor an advocacy assistance program. Executive directors or the senior elected official of each of the thirty-three statewide associations of not-for-profit nursing homes (American Association of Homes for the Aged) were reached, as were those for the forty-eight state chapters of the primarily proprietary nursing home associations of the American Health Care Association. For each of these respondent groups, therefore, the sampling constituted universal categories.

In the case of state-level citizens organizations that specialize in advocacy for the institutionalized aged, a purposive sample was recruited. State commissioners on aging were asked to identify three such organizations. The first organization on the list was then included in the sample if it was not a direct spon-

sor of the ombudsman program or a chapter of the National
Retired Teachers Association-American Association of Retired
Persons (NRTA-AARP). If the first organization listed was inappropriate due to these criteria, the second organization was
included in the sample, and so on. Forty-two states provided
such lists.

For the remainder, citizen advocacy organizatons for the
aged were selected from lists provided by the National Citizens' Coalition for Nursing Home Reform. A grand total of
forty-six such state community action interest groups for the
elderly was thus identified and contact made.

Following mail distribution of the survey instruments, sample sizes were adjusted in accordance with supplementary information received about the proposed samples. Due to vacancies in a few positions or to other factors causing questionnaires
to be returned but not completed, a final revised total for each
category was established. Of the corrected grand total of 358
potential respondents, 265 (74 percent) completed the questionnaires.

A look at the distribution of respondent groups in the sample according to four demographic criteria reveals relatively
equal representation by each of the categories. The distributions were viewed according to region, state elderly population, state nursing home population, and the nursing home
bed/elder population ratio.

REGION

The distribution of individual respondent categories in four
geographic regions—Northeast, North Central, South, and
West—is quite similar to the summary breakdown by region:
a quarter each in the West and North Central regions, a third
in the South, and a sixth in the Northeast. Slight variations
were noted. In particular, the relatively higher number of
commissioners of welfare in the Northeast and few in the
North Central region; the greater proportion of nonprofit
nursing home association respondents from the South and

fewer from the West; and the relatively greater representation of proprietary nursing home associations from the West and correspondingly fewer from the South. On the whole, however, the distribution of each category according to the regional criterion may be said to be much the same.

The distribution of respondent categories by state elderly population shows similar uniformity across the categories:

Less than 250,000 (small)
250,000 to 499,999 (low-medium)
500,000 to 999,999 (high-medium)
1,000,000 or more (large).

The entire respondent pool was represented by about one third from states with small elderly populations, one third from states with low-medium elderly populations, and one sixth each from those with high-medium and large elderly populations. A review of individual categories reveals similar distributions except for the following minor variations: commissioners of welfare had higher representation from the states with a small elderly population and lower representation for high-medium state populations of elderly; nonprofit nursing home associations that responded were less likely to be from states with small elderly populations, and more likely to be from low-medium state elderly populations. In general, however, similar trends may be cited for the distribution of all categories in regard to the elderly population of the states.

The states' nursing home populations were derived from the 1978 National Master Facility Inventory of Nursing Homes and Hospitals.[1] They were divided into three categories: small (less than 10,000), medium (10,000 to 49,999), and large (50,000

or more). Overall respondents' distribution by this demographic variable indicates that states with a small nursing home
population accounted for about one third of the respondents,
states with a medium nursing home patient population slightly
more than half the respondents, and states with a large population less than one-sixth of the respondents. Once again, the
respondent categories showed similar distributions, except for
three minor variations: legal services developers were overre-
presented in the medium population range and underrepre-
sented in the large population grouping; welfare commissioners were more likely than the overall distribution to be from
states with small nursing home populations and less likely to
be from states with a medium-sized population in nursing
homes; and nonprofit nursing home associations reversed the
trend set by the welfare commissioners. The overall distribution, nevertheless, shows a uniformity of response rates for
each respondent category when divided by the states' nursing
home population.

NURSING HOME BED/ELDER POPULATION RATIOS

Finally, the distribution of each category by level of nursing
home beds per 1,000 individuals aged 65 years and over in
each state showed trends similar to the overall breakdown. Four
levels of bed/population ratios were determined:

Small bed/population ratio (20–39 beds)
Low-medium bed/population ratio (40–59 beds)
High-medium bed/population ratio (60–79 beds)
Large bed/population ratio (80–111 beds).

For the entire respondent sample, states with small
bed/population ratios accounted for 16 percent of the respondents, states with a low-medium bed/population ratio 44
percent of the respondents, states with a high-medium
bed/population 22 percent of the respondents, and states with
a large bed/population ratio 18 percent of the respondents.

When viewed by individual study group, it was seen that no group, except for the commissioners of welfare, varied by more than 5 percent from the overall distribution.

Thus, in sum, the distribution of the eight respondent categories in the study sample along four relevant demographic variables reflects a strong similarity. While identical distributions are not to be expected from samples whose response is determined by self-choice, the generally uniform trends obtained from the respondent categories make comparisons between them valid and meaningful. Furthermore, low chi-squares achieved in the cross-tabulation of each demographic variable with the study groups verifies the lack of significant variation between the study groups. The study sample is therefore considered to be a representative one, given the high response rate, and an internally comparable one, based upon the uniform distributions of each category of respondents.

Survey Instruments

Structured survey questionnaires were developed for the two major groupings of respondents: state nursing home ombudsmen and the long-term care network.

Ombudsman questionnaire. This instrument aimed at gathering base-line data on the following aspects of nursing home ombudsman programs in each state:

Descriptive/historical
Personal involvement of state ombudsmen
Role/function of ombudsman position
Factors determining efficacy
Interorganizational relations
Staffing patterns
Organizational location and accountability
State/local relations
Recruitment/retention of volunteers
Effectiveness
Scope

Power to intervene
Program issues/problems.

The instrument consisted of thirty-nine question areas and required approximately one hour to complete. Both descriptive and prescriptive responses were differentially solicited by selected questions. A mix of open-end and closed-end/check-off question formats was employed.

Network questionnaire. A shorter version of the above questionnaire was designed to maximize receipt of a wide range of perceptions about the ombudsman program. Questions focused largely on:

Role/function of ombudsman program
Factors determining efficacy
Interorganizational relations
Organizational location and accountability
Effectiveness
Scope
Power to intervene
Program issues/problems
Value of ombudsman program.

The network survey instrument consisted of eighteen question areas and required less than half an hour to complete. The exclusive use of closed-end and check-off questions was intended to elicit a high rate of response. Both national survey questionnaires were pretested with a select group of federal, state, and local representatives knowledgeable in nursing home ombudsman issues but not included in the respondent samples.

Semistructured interviewing guides were developed for utilization during selected on-site field visits of state ombudsman programs. They were designed to obtain detailed descriptions of program process reflective of service organization and delivery and not obtainable through the mailed survey strategy. Issues of central importance considered during field interviews included the detailed specification of program-specific methodology and the description of daily service flow patterns in the areas of: recruitment, orientation, training, supervision/case management, administration and policy, outreach/publicity, record-keeping/data collection (accountability patterns), and interorganizational relationships.

A purposive sample of state ombudsman programs was chosen for the on-site interviewing. Criteria utilized in the selection of this study group included both programmatic and geographic factors. Preliminary review of state ombudsman reports enabled the researchers to identify the state nursing home ombudsman programs with major differences in program structure, staffing, focus, and scope.

Subsequent pilot interviews with the office of the federal ombudsman and with the National Citizens' Coalition for Nursing Home Reform helped clarify state program differences. The final choice of state programs reflected, therefore, a range of possible program prototypes, and a geographically diverse sample. The states visited were California, Oregon, Florida, Georgia, Minnesota, Michigan, Connecticut, New Jersey, and New York.

Finally, additional unobtrusive data in the form of ombudsman program reports and publications were solicited. Material was received from thirty-one state nursing home ombudsman programs, 60.8 percent of those approached.

Data Collection

The first wave of structured questionnaires were mailed in April 1981 to 396 individuals in the eight respondent categories. The response rate for the first mailing was 55.3 percent. A second mailing and follow-up phone calls took place in May, achieving the final response rate of 74.0 percent. The on-site visits were carried out during the summer and early fall of 1981.

Data Analysis

Descriptive statistics, frequency distribution, and cross-tabulations were applied as well as chi-square, *T*-tests, and one-way analysis of variance. Factor analysis was also employed for a selected set of variables.

A major vehicle for data analysis was the application of scales tapping a range of perceptions. Four scales were incorporated from the preceding New York City study. These instruments (role perception scale, program power scale, perceived effectiveness scale, and perceived impact scale) were again found to be internally reliable and hence were employed in the analysis. Two new scales were created for the national study as well. These indices (issue effectiveness scale and complaint effectiveness scale) were also found to be internally reliable. Further information concerning scale construction and reliability, as well as the findings derived from the various statistical analyses and field visits, are presented and discussed in chapters 4 to 7 as well as Appendix A and B.

CHAPTER FOUR

The Ombudsman and the Complaint Grievance Process

Nursing home ombudsman programs are mandated by law. Review of individual state reports collected during the study reveals, however, that each state has gone its own way in deciding upon the organizational format and the type of legal supports for this newly developed service. Content analysis of the state material was hindered by the variation in its scope and quality. Some reports were limited to brief memoranda while others covered volumes of sophisticated survey information. Insofar as this heterogeneity conspired against the generalization of findings, the authors chose, in addition, to identify distinctive prototypes among state ombudsman programs, using information about their organizational design, legal status, and mode of operation as differentiating criteria.

Additional variations were noticed in the location of the ombudsman program within each state government system as well as the extent of centralization of its operation, the volunteer or salaried status of state and local ombudsmen, the right of access to nursing home facilities, the association with other program networks, and the actual volume of ombudsman activity. Other more subtle differences suggested from the state literature include as well variations in program orientation toward the ombudsman's role and function. The focus of the role may be described as ranging in concentration on licensure, abuse of patients, patients' rights, and interpersonal relations. The ombudsman's function oscillates between a consensus-collaborative orientation and an advocacy-contest perspective, with a therapy-oriented function in a somewhat ancillary position alongside the other two.

The comparison may commence at the point of the program's administrative placement within a state's government or its service network. Nearly half of the state reports noted the location of the ombudsman program in independent divisions on aging. About one third are in state departments of human resources, health and social services, economic security, and public welfare. One tenth found the ombudsman program under the aegis of a public executive (governor or, as in the case of Washington, D.C. the mayor). Two states reported their nursing home ombudsman programs were contracted to private or voluntary organizations at the administrative level, and only one, New Jersey, reported the unique establishment of a state ombudsman for the institutionalized aged and a department of the public advocate through which the nursing home ombudsman can resort to litigation. Table 4.1 summarizes the administrative affiliation of the programs.

Table 4.1
Administrative Location of Nursing Home Ombudsman Programs at the State Level

Location	N	Percent
Independent governmental division on aging	24	46.2
Department of human services (health or welfare)	17	32.7
Office of the chief executive (governor, or mayor of D.C.)	6	11.5
Contracted to a citizens' organization	2	3.8
Other	3	5.8
TOTAL	52	100.0

As observed, one third of nursing home ombudsman programs are located in departments that may well have other procedural dealings with nursing homes, such as licensing or reimbursement arrangements. This raises some question as to the presumed objectivity, independence, and impartiality that are imputed to the ombudsman in the literature.

The degree of centralization of the nursing home ombudsman program also varies from state to state. Roughly a third of the states indicated centralized patterns of ombudsman service delivery, while two thirds operate through varying forms of regional delivery structures. In some cases the centralized nature of the program may be related to the small size of the respective state (Delaware and Hawaii, for example), but in others, like New Jersey, it may well be a function of its structure, fashioned along classical ombudsman lines. Similarly, the decentralized versions of the nursing home ombudsman program show variations that go beyond the size of the state nursing home resident population.

While almost all the states report the presence of a salaried ombudsman development specialist, as called for in the Older Americans Act amendments of 1978, the status of the ombudsman at the regional level also varies among different states. Ombudsman services at the point of delivery may be characterized by salaried professional ombudsman services, a mix of salaried professionals and volunteers, or volunteer activity only. Examples of these three possible patterns are:

1. Salaried professional ombudsmen: Montana, which contracted out its nursing home ombudsman program to the Montana Legal Service Association. Twelve part-time paralegals worked on a salaried basis as regional ombudsmen throughout the state.
2. Mix of salaried ombudsmen and volunteers: Indiana, whose nursing home ombudsman program consisted of statewide ombudsman coordinators, seven salaried area ombudsmen, and fifty volunteers.
3. Volunteer ombudsmen only: Florida, with a network of area committees that serve as the respective areas' regional nursing home ombudsmen, and report to a state committee and a statewide ombudsman.

Survey findings indicated that seventeen programs (42.5 percent) were composed almost entirely of paid staff; seven programs (17.5 percent) relied largely on paid staff and some volunteers; three programs (7.5 percent) were staffed equally by volunteers and paid staff; nine programs (22.5 percent) depended mostly on volunteers, with some paid staff; and four programs (10.0 percent) were composed almost entirely of volunteer staff.

The availability of mandated access by ombudsmen to nursing home facilities was explicitly mentioned in less than a third of the reports. Table 4.2 summarizes the extent of legal powers granted to state programs.

Table 4.2
The Attainment of Statutory Powers as Reported by State Nursing Home Ombudsman Programs (1981)

Statutory Powers		*Yes*		*No*		*Total*
	N	*Percent*	*N*	*Percent*	*N*	*Percent*
Authority to change decisions made in nursing homes	4	10.5	34	89.5	38	100.0
Authority to enforce decisions made in nursing homes	4	10.5	34	89.5	38	100.0
Access to all nursing homes	20	52.6	18	47.4	38	100.0
Access to patient records	14	36.8	24	63.2	38	100.0
Legislative/legal authority in performing their function	13	34.2	25	65.8	38	100.0

The access question may be divided into two parts: whether there exists mandated entry, and if so, for whom.

The first point offers three possibilities: the lack of a state nursing home ombudsman bill to mandate access; the presence of a state nursing home ombudsman bill, but one that lacks the legal right of access; and the presence of a state nursing home ombudsman bill that does mandate access. Variations on this theme include bills that have been proposed but were not enacted at the time of the study.

Representative of the first possibility is Arizona, which, lacking a specific piece of legislation authorizing a nursing home ombudsman, operated its program as part of adult protective services in the Department of Economic Security. Departmental staff in the local offices acted as ombudsmen for institutionalized adults within the parameters of protective services, but did not have mandated access to facilities.

Utah, Montana, and Minnesota represented the second possibility, states that did not have mandated access to facilities but had nursing home ombudsman programs in operation. The status of nursing home ombudsman legislation in each of these states was not clearly articulated in their reports, but they presumably reflected variations at the second level of mandated access put forward here.

Finally, examples of the third possibility—legislated access for nursing home ombudsmen—are North and South Carolina. The difference between those two programs leads to the next, related, point: mandated access for whom?

In North Carolina the legislation provided for the mandated access of the state's 425 volunteers operating through 75 volunteer committees. South Carolina's legislation, on the other hand, mandated access for the state nursing home ombudsman only, despite the fact that the state has a network of volunteer ombudsmen as well. In other states, the respective mix of salaried versus volunteer ombudsmen, with mandated access or not, and at which level, sets the stage for differing expressions of the nursing home ombudsmen program at the point of service delivery.

State nursing home ombudsman programs differ in other aspects as well. Some of the programs are relatively freestanding while others are part of a larger advocacy assistance program or other service network. Four states (Arkansas, Montana, Minnesota, and Massachusetts) and Puerto Rico specifically mentioned an association between the nursing home ombudsman program and the larger advocacy assistance for older Americans program. Washington, D.C., saw its nursing home ombudsman program as part of an overall long-term care system. Arizona viewed its protective services-based ombudsmen as part of a legal advisory network, and in South Dakota they were seen as part of long-term care protective services. The characteristics of the network with which the nursing home ombudsman program is associated take on greater relevance when considering the next point: the range of populations served by the network.

The nursing home ombudsman program is ostensibly geared toward the needs of the institutionalized elderly. When viewed in the larger network framework, however, there are two possible directions in which the larger network tends to focus: serving all the elderly, whether institutionalized or not; or serving all long-term care patients, whether elderly or not. Examples of the former are Arkansas and Minnesota, while an example of the latter is South Dakota. Table 4.3 reflects the reported trends in the scope of serviced populations.

Table 4.3
Varying Scope of Nursing Home Ombudsman Serviced Populations

Serviced Populations	N	Percent
The LTCOP* serves only elderly in the LTC facilities	14	33.3
The LTCOP serves all elderly, whether in LTC facilities or not	7	16.7
The LTCOP serves everyone in LTC facilities whether elderly or not	20	47.6
Other	1	2.4
TOTAL	42	100.0

*Long-term care ombudsman program

In terms of the volume of complaints that nursing home ombudsmen are asked to deal with, only fourteen states provided information that could be viewed numerically, and even among these states the reporting was far from uniform. In addition, the absolute numbers taken by themselves have little significance without knowledge of the overall institutionalized population in each state, or of the nature of the complaints included in the reporting.

Unfortunately, data did not allow for the computation of informative ratios, such as the relationship of the number of complaints to the size of the patients' population, or the relationship of the number of complaints serviced to the number of active ombudsman volunteers. In only one report, that of Connecticut, was any such ratio indicated. In Connecticut the nursing home ombudsman program calls for one "advocate" per 100 patients. Such a ratio of ombudsmen, patients, and complaints remains a critical area for exploration that still needs to be done if the state nursing home ombudsman programs are to be validly and reliably compared.

A final distinction relates to variations in program focus. Four such orientations in program primacy have been identified and may be summarized as follows:

1. *Focus on abuse of patients.* Ombudsman activity that responds primarily to reports of abuse or neglect of patients in the long-term care facility, such as striking patients or the use of unwarranted constraints, overmedication, and purposeful neglect
2. *Focus on licensure.* Activity aimed at bringing violations of the required standards of the long-term care facility to light and initiating corrective procedures. Documented examples include fire hazards, the illegal placement of beds in basements or attics, and structural deficiencies.
3. *Focus on patients' rights.* These activities aim at guaranteeing patients' rights, such as the private use of the telephone, the right to visitation, and the safeguarding of one's belongings. Many states have such personal rights already enumerated in a patients' bill of rights. This statement serves as a framework for this category of program emphasis by nursing home ombudsmen.
4. *Interpersonal focus.* The least defined of the respective program foci, this concentrates upon the friendly visiting aspect of the ombudsman contact. Such activity may also deal with social relations among patients or patients' relations with their families and friends.

Review of the state reports indicated that while the four ombudsman program foci are not mutually exclusive, state programs tend to lean more decisively toward a given one as their preferred model. The focus on abuse of patients is most prevalent in states that operate the nursing home ombudsman program under the aegis of adult protective services. In South

Dakota eligibility requirements make the receipt of ombuds- man services conditional upon being "in need of protection." Arizona similarly operates its nursing home ombudsman pro- gram through adult protective services. On the other hand, the focus on abuse of patients is not limited to nonmandated programs per se. For example, South Carolina and Georgia, each with a legislatively based nursing home ombudsman, in- dicated in their reports some tendency to focus on abuse of patients and its amelioration.

Licensure-focused activities are present to varying degrees in most states. Those with specialized investigative personnel, like New Jersey, would be more likely to emphasize this ap- proach. A focus on patients' rights is similarly considered to be widely adopted, but varies to the degree that states have legislation anchoring the preservation of patients' rights in law. In addition, the extent of the focus on patients' rights seems to vary along with the extent of general advocacy activities car- ried out by larger advocacy assistance networks, within which some nursing home ombudsman programs operate.

Finally, the interpersonal focus is found to be openly es- poused in only a small minority of the state programs. A prime example is Utah, which lacks mandated authority for its nurs- ing home ombudsman program. In that state, fourteen local ombudsmen (resource aids) work in five nursing homes as friendly visitors. Included among their tasks is leading sing- alongs with the residents.

Program Prototypes

This overview of the nursing home ombudsman programs, based upon the state reports, would not be complete without an in-depth examination of the programs in selected states, each representing a sufficiently different prototype to warrant specific attention. The state nursing home ombudsman pro- grams to be discussed are those in Connecticut, New Jersey, Florida, Massachusetts, and Michigan. A brief review of aspects of the New York State program is also included because it constitutes an eclectic effort that incorporates elements of all five prototypical programs.

Connecticut

The Nursing Home Ombudsman Office in the state of Connecticut is a project of the state's Department of Aging, as prescribed in the legislative bill creating the office in 1977, P.A. 77-575.[1] The act calls for the Commissioner on Aging to appoint a state ombudsman and five regional ombudsmen. Volunteer patient advocates at the local level are appointed by the state ombudsman and serve, after a ninety-day trial period, without compensation other than reimbursement for expenses.

The act sets forth the following duties for the state ombudsman:

1. To establish program policies and procedures for handling complaints from patients, families, employees of nursing home facilities, and the general public.
2. To carry out established policies and procedures
3. To work with appropriate organizations to clarify and resolve complaints
4. To provide information to such organizations as requested
5. To collect data for research and analysis and make recommendations for policy and program changes
6. To identify and document problems affecting a large segment of the nursing home facility population and communicate these problems to groups and agencies who can deal with such problems
7. To publicize the ombudsman program, its purposes, and mode of operation
8. To submit legislative recommendations to the general assembly.

The regional ombudsmen perform similar functions in their respective locales. The heart of the program, however, is in the use of trained patients' advocates, assigned on the basis of one advocate per 100 patients. Thus one advocate may cover a few small homes while a larger scale long-term care facility may have several advocates. The advocate is the first-line service deliverer whose job is to receive complaints and problems from such sources as patients, administration, staff, family, and friends. The act creating the Nursing Home Ombudsman Office prescribes duties for the patients' advocates identical to those set forth for state ombudsmen. It adds the responsibilities for:

1. Facilitating private legal action for patients if necessary
2. Assuring that the patients' bill of rights is posted and that all the provisions in the bill are adhered to
3. Aiding patients with the administrative aspects of transfers and discharges and aiding in ensuring that patients are satisfied with the management of their financial affairs.

The first priority of these advocates is to attempt to resolve a particular problem within the nursing home facility. If problems arise that require referrals to other agencies, they are acted upon by the regional ombudsman. Thus, despite the title of "advocate" the locally based patients' advocates of Connecticut first attempt to work through collaborative processes; failing that, they pass on the responsibility and follow-up to the salaried regional ombudsman.

It is significant to note that both salaried ombudsmen and volunteer patient advocates have mandated access to all nursing home facilities—refusal to cooperate results in a penalty for the facility—and access to all "relevant public records." Records that are confidential to a patient may be viewed if the ombudsman or advocate is given written consent by the patient or by his/her caretaker. Furthermore, the nursing home ombudsman legislation is strengthened by Connecticut state law, which mandates specific categories of people (administration and staff of nursing homes, social workers, nurses and doctors) to report to the ombudsman office, suspected abuse, neglect, exploitation, or abandonment of a nursing home resident. The law further provides for protection from liability for filers of complaints, be they patients or staff.

In reviewing the first two years of the program's functioning, certain trends may be identified.[2] The program attracted 175 volunteer advocates who ranged in age from twenty-one to eighty-plus years, with backgrounds varying from high school education to masters' degrees in health and social welfare related areas. According to the 1978 annual report:

> The majority of problems received and investigated dealt with quality of care in the facilities such as short staffing, call bells not being answered, patients wet and not being changed, no ambulation of patients, patients not being fed, unauthorized personnel dispensing medication, accidents not being reported, lack of supervision, lack of training of aides, indifference and rudeness by staff.[3]

A second significant complaint category was the mishandling of patients' personal funds by sources outside the long-term care facility, as for example by families, conservators, representative payees, or people with power of attorney. This repeated problem coupled with the recurring loss of patients' personal belongings in the nursing home led to the establishment of guidelines and forms for dealing with them by the ombudsman office. Obstacles which have impeded problem resolution, on the other hand, include such factors outside the facilities as inadequacies of the public health code and regulations of the Department of Income Maintenance.

Thus, in sum, the Connecticut nursing home ombudsman program represents the statute-rooted, regionally structured, and locally based collaborative ombudsman services that are delivered by volunteer advocates. While sharing some general characteristics, the Connecticut program differs in a significant way from that of the New Jersey ombudsman for the institutionalized elderly.

New Jersey

The New Jersey nursing home ombudsman program may be traced back to 1975 when the state became a recipient of an AoA discretionary grant to promote and develop state and area ombudsman services. The present form of the program and its mark of distinction, however, derive from the creation of the New Jersey State Office of the Ombudsman for the Institutionalized Elderly (NJSA 52:27G-1 to 16, approved September 29, 1977). The office became functional in May of 1978 with the appointment of a former state senator as ombudsman.

The office is described by the incumbent as the "strongest" such office in the nation, whose primacy is in its advocacy role for the institutionalized elderly.[4] The structure and function of the office bear testimony to its advocate nature. The ombudsman office is officially allocated to the Department of Community Affairs for administrative purposes, but it is independent of supervision or control by that department. At the same time, the Office of the Ombudsman maintains what it terms "a contractual relationship with the New Jersey Department of the Public Advocate to facilitate the provision of legal services by and for this office."[5] Ultimately, the ombudsman for the institutionalized elderly is directly responsible to the governor, as befits the model of the executive ombudsman. A secondary role of the New Jersey office is to work with the state and county offices on aging to recruit and provide back-up support to ombudsman community volunteer groups, and to do the same in the private sector among voluntary organizations. The peripheral nature and status of these tasks, however, are underscored by the following description of the ombudsman's activities which stress

> investigations, negotiations, conducting hearings with subpoena authority, bringing suit for injunctive relief, civil damages and . . . [enforcing any of the power enumerated in the Ombudsman enabling legislation, NJSA 52:27G-1 et seq.[6]

The legal authority of the office, which includes subpoena power, the right to litigate, and the right to hold public hearings, backs up the adversarial-advocacy focus of the New Jersey Ombudsman for the Institutionalized Elderly. The highlights cited in the first year report similarly underscore the advocacy approach: the initiation of grand jury proceedings concerning abuse of patients, and the resulting indictment of a facility's owner and revocation of his license; the curtailment of admissions to facilities because of noncompliance in the correction of deficiencies; input in the formulation of standards for licensure; and the drafting of major state regulations.

Complaints are received through the mail, by telephone, or through a hot-line operator. They are then turned over to the state ombudsman's investigatory staff, consisting of five registered nurses and three former law enforcement officers. Investigatory visits to facilities follow the receipt of complaints and may be carried out during the night shift as well as during the day shift. These visits are always unannounced.

In sum, the New Jersey nursing home ombudsman program is unique in the presence of a state-level executive ombudsman whose power and focus place this program at the adversarial end of the program strategy continuum, far afield from Connecticut's more collaborative approach. A third variation in the program structure, one that falls between the two models previously discussed, may be found in Florida.

Florida

The Florida nursing home ombudsman program dates back to 1975 when the state legislature created a system of citizen committees "to serve as advocates on behalf of nursing home residents and their families."[7] The system of one statewide and eleven district committees was founded to augment the protection of nursing home residents' rights, in view of the failure of regulatory agencies and the nursing home industry to do so. The legislation confers upon the statewide committee the following duties:

1. To help establish and coordinate the district ombudsman committees
2. To serve as an appellate body in receiving from the district ombudsman committees complaints not resolved at the district level
3. To develop procedures for eliciting, receiving, responding to, and resolving complaints made by, and on behalf of, nursing home residents
4. To elicit and coordinate state, local, and voluntary organizational assistance for the purpose of improving the care received by nursing home residents.

The district ombudsman committees were in turn charged to:

1. Serve as third-party mechanisms for protecting the health, safety, welfare, and civil and human rights of nursing home residents
2. Discover, investigate, and determine the existence of abuse and neglect in the nursing home
3. Elicit, receive, respond to, and resolve complaints made by or on behalf of nursing home residents
4. Review rules and regulations relating to nursing homes for their effect on residents' rights.

The district ombudsman committees are granted statutorily based rights of access to nursing homes and to Medicaid patients' personal property and money accounts "pursuant to an investigation to obtain information regarding a specific complaint or problem."[8]

Most unique in the Florida ombudsman committee system is the legally predetermined composition of the committees, both state-wide and district based. The legislation calls for the appointment of one medical doctor whose practice includes a substantial number of geriatric patients; one registered nurse; one nursing home administrator; one licensed pharmacist; one dietician; nursing home residents or representative consumer advocates for nursing home residents (2 for statewide committee, 5 each for district committees); one attorney; and one professional social worker.[9]

The committee members are appointed for two-year terms, and members may serve two consecutive terms. All vacancies are filled by the governor, who may declare as vacant the term of any member who misses three consecutive regular meetings without cause. The members of the committees receive no compensation, but are reimbursed for travel expenses. Thus the ombudsman committees invoke the need for civic duty among individuals in the long-term care community.

At the time of the study, the committees were officially in the office of the governor, but administratively assigned to the Department of Health and Rehabilitative Services. As stated in the yearly report of 1978, "this structure raises the conflict of interest issue as the committees are administered by the same department which licenses, inspects and regulates nursing homes."[10] The State Ombudsman Committee has, therefore, called for more direct links with the governor's office.

The 1981 state report indicates that most complaints in the 1980–81 fiscal year were received in the area of patient care, followed by administration and staff-related complaints.[11]

In summary, the Florida nursing home ombudsman program has attempted to capitalize upon the advantages of both the volunteer-based Connecticut patients' advocate structure and the New Jersey ombudsman's executive approach. It seems, however, that in attempting both, the program has not marshaled enough authority. The district committee members may meet only once a month while the statewide committee is required to meet only once in a quarter (although it may choose to convene more often). The limitations of this system that have been alluded to so far are reflected in the state committee's expressed support for the development of a department or office of public advocacy in Florida.

Massachusetts

Massachusetts began its ombudsman services for the institutionalized elderly in the second year of the U.S. Department of Health, Education, and Welfare demonstration project period. It represents the model of a nursing home ombudsman program that has become part of a larger advocacy network, serving the elderly in the community as well as those in long-term care facilities, and addressing issues of relevance to elders more generally. The strengthened community focus and the reliance upon locally based volunteer organizations where possible serve as additional factors which distinguish the Massachusetts ombudsman program.

Structurally, the older Americans advocacy assistance program serves as an umbrella program for both the nursing home ombudsman and legal service developer projects, and constitutes in itself a division within the advocacy unit of the Massachusetts Department of Elder Affairs. The older Americans advocacy assistance program serves as a clearinghouse for information and referral in regard to long-term care issues, consumer protection, medical insurance, public benefits programs, and legal concerns of the elderly. The central office staff receives and resolves complaints while simultaneously seeking to foster local capacities, through organization, development, and training, to provide advocacy to the elderly.

The goals of the program include:

1. Improving the quality of care, life, and environment in long-term care facilities
2. Eliminating discrimination against those who are publicly assisted
3. Assisting in placement of "hard-to-place" nursing home patients
4. Channeling complaints through the state departments of public health and public welfare, the attorney general's office, the Rate Setting Commission, and the Department of Mental Health
5. Assisting community based elderly, especially in consumer and legal affairs

6. Providing information and referral regarding any aspect of long-term care, public benefit programs, and Medicare
7. Assisting development of legal services for the elderly
8. Distributing timely information on affairs of the elderly
9. Developing a network of trained volunteers and coordinating training programs
10. Working with state agencies and the legislature to upgrade the quality of life for all elders.[12]

The state program encourages a locally based focus, but the state office remains as a more frequent recipient of complaints relating to patient care and to professional services than the local programs. When combining state- and local-level reporting statistics for a recent year, the complaints most often raised were: (1) lack of cleanliness of the facility; (2) food; (3) staffing and professional services; (4) patients' care; (5) patients' rights; (6) missing items; and (7) financial concerns. Similarly, the problems which were most frequently reported involved Medicare and Medicaid claims, financial problems, guardianship/conservatorship issues, and Social Security payments.

Thus, as the description of the complaints gathered in the Massachusetts nursing home ombudsman program shows, this state's program is similar in content and context to other nursing home ombudsman programs. Its uniqueness lies in the diversity of local programs that make up the statewide advocacy network, and "a definite shift toward complaint and problem resolution at the local level."[13]

Michigan

This program is of significance because its headquarters were initially not in Michigan, but in Washington, D.C. This was because the program operated under the auspices of a voluntary organization, the National Council of Senior Citizens (NCSC), and not by the state in which it functioned. Subsequently, the state nursing home ombudsman program was contracted to Citizens for Better Care (CBC), a consumer advisory organization in Michigan. Thus this nursing home ombudsman program presented a final option for consideration, a strictly voluntary model of ombudsman services, from administration through service delivery.

The program was at first composed of varying components operating with relative independence one from another. The national office focused upon what has been termed in other state reports "issues advocacy," and specifically upon federal legislation and regulations. The state office dealt primarily with state policies, legislation, and regulations related to long-term care, while the local offices concentrated upon complaint resolution. The Detroit local office was contracted to CBC, which later assumed responsibility for the entire statewide program.

CBC was founded in 1969, even before the initiation of the nursing home ombudsman concept, as a member-based consumer organization concerned with the improvement of nursing homes. It has since grown to include all problems of the elderly and the health of the general public as well. Under the auspices of the 1978 amendments to the Older Americans Act, expanding the nursing home ombudsman program, CBC took on its statewide role, and subsequently became the recipient of an expanded grant award from the Commission on Aging for its long-term care ombudsman project. It is pertinent, therefore, to look at the ombudsman role developed by CBC.

The ombudsman thus envisioned is a resident advocate volunteer whose roles are spelled out in the *Organizers Manual for Nursing Home Ombudsmen,* published by CBC in 1976:

> The resident advocate volunteer would have multiple roles. Their primary role is to act as a spokesman for residents by communicating their concerns to the appropriate staff members in a home and see to it that the problem is resolved. The advocate serves as a link and mediator between residents and staff, between residents and community/government agencies and between residents and family members. The advocate also serves as teacher in using his knowledge of rules, regulations and procedures to assist residents, relatives, and frequently nursing home staff, in understanding some of the very technical requirements of the field.

In addition, the advocate also observes conditions in the home, investigates problems to determine their validity, records these problems, and works with the staff to ensure that these issues are responded to positively. The advocates report to CBC to inform us of the homes' progress and to assist them and the home in resolving concerns. Also the advocate and the CBC office support staff serve to motivate the home to provide quality care, as well as serving as a resource whenever feasible.

The advocates will visit with residents, listen to their concerns and assist them through personal contact to obtain solutions to their problems by directing them to appropriate staff members or, if necessary, outside agencies.[14]

Thus CBC favored a cooperative relationship between ombudsman and facilities, providing "a person who will devote himself entirely to listening and responding to concerns of residents."[15] This, in turn, was said to benefit the level of services, save time, and contribute to improved community relations. It may also provide "ongoing feedback to the facility about the concerns of their residents."[16] The voluntary nature of the ombudsman sponsor was seen as a facilitating agent in the implementation of the suggested ombudsman roles.

The volunteer nature of the program's organization has drawn certain criticisms, however. A 1975 report by AoA's Nursing Home Interests staff assessing the nursing home ombudsman demonstration program noted that the early NCSC/Michigan project exhibited lack of coordination among its varying units, with the national office in Washington unable to provide effective leadership to the state and local units. Furthermore, the voluntary organization status occasionally caused limited access to government agencies. Finally, much of the project rested upon CBC's preestablished reputation which was generally effective, but had seemingly alienated the nursing home industry to some degree through its more adversarial and litigative methods and actions.[17]

As in other states' ombudsman programs, the Michigan project pinpointed ongoing problems in long-term care. They included the disregard of patients' rights, restricted Medicaid coverage, chronic noncompliance with codes and the need for improved monitoring by the regulatory agencies.[18]

The original NCSC/Michigan nursing home ombudsman program thus approximated other collaboratively based programs, but it tended to rely more upon such strategy due to its voluntary organizational status. The more recent version of Michigan's nursing home ombudsman program under the auspices of CBC, on the other hand, eschews the collaborative mode in favor of a contest orientation, despite its voluntary organizational status.

New York

The New York State long-term care ombudsman program came into being early in 1977 and is housed within the AoA State Office for the Aging. The State Office for the Aging was deemed the appropriate sponsor due to its traditional "advocate-for-the-elderly" orientation as well as the absence of any responsibility actually to survey facilities, issue licenses, or set reimbursement rates.

The first local programs began in Ulster and Greene counties. Prior to and during this time, the Community Council of Greater New York developed both a model plan for ombudsman service organization and a training/design curriculum for the program. The model plan emphasized three major components:

1. *A "back-up" agency.* Responsible for program coordination at the local level; recruitment and supervision of citizen ombudsmen; establishing linkages with public agencies for resolution of unresolved complaints
2. *Citizen ombudsmen.* Volunteers, trained in patient advocacy, who regularly visit nursing home patients—the outreach arm of the program
3. *State nursing home ombudsman.* Charged to initiate and coordinate local programs; develop training curricula for ombudsmen and their supervisors; provide technical assistance to back-up agencies; and serve as spokespersons for patients at the state level.[19]

The basic approach to complaint resolution in New York State has been through informed mediation and conciliation.

Attempts are first made to resolve complaints in-house. Only when this fails are complaints referred to the back-up agency; then, if necessary, to the state agency having jurisdiction. Included here are the Office of Health Systems Management of the State Department of Health, Division of Adult Residential Care of the State Department of Social Services, the special prosecutor, and local supervisory agencies such as county offices of social services.[20]

The State Office for the Aging focuses primarily on generic issues. Whereas local programs document specific grievances, the staff of the State Office for the Aging identify systemic types of complaints that affect a group of individuals rather than individual patients. The eight general categories of concern are: (1) quality of care; (2) food/nutrition; (3) administration; (4) environment/sanitation; (5) patients' rights; (6) abuse; (7) financial; and (8) other.

The first annual state report for New York State indicated that quality-of-care grievances were handled most often (27.3 percent), followed by food/nutrition (21.8 percent), administration (17.6 percent), and environmental issues (10.9 percent). Less often handled were financial, patients' rights, and abuse issues. It is interesting to note that local programs, as a group, have been most successful in resolving complaints of abuse although the total handled was quite small during the reporting period (October 1, 1977—September 30, 1978). Ombudsman were least successful in resolving certain other complaints, including family disputes and grievances against local agencies such as the Medicaid office.

New York State volunteer ombudsmen have extended their responsibilities beyond efforts to resolve nursing home complaints. The following list is a sampling of the kinds of parallel activities in which ombudsmen have been involved.

1. A local veterans' organization wanted a list of vets residing in the facility. With the help of facility staff, the ombudsman put a list together and sent it to the vets' organizations.
2. A relative of a patient makes contact with the ombudsman to find out how the patient was doing. The ombudsman helped the patient dictate a letter to the relative.

3. An ombudsman was invited by residents to help conduct a residents' council meeting.
4. The ombudsman reacted to a resident having a heart attack: helped dress the resident, called for an ambulance, and stayed with the panicstricken resident until the ambulance arrived. This was in a small adult home where only two aides were on duty.
5. A patient asked the ombudsman to find out how a patient could become a U.S. citizen. The ombudsman contacted a Congressman's office and helped the patient complete forms.[21]

In essence, ombudsmen throughout New York State, as in other areas of the United States, perform functions beyond those of complaint resolution.

In examining how ombudsman programs operate, special attention must be given to the complaint grievance process. Most of this information is primarily drawn from the New York City ombudsman study. It may be recalled that the researchers conducted more direct field observations in this initial phase of research.

Organizational Location

Responsibility for implementation of the ombudsman program in New York City has resided with a voluntary, city-wide planning and consumer participation organization. The Community Council of Greater New York has traditionally been identified with the development and promotion of social policy research and information in the field of human services. A definite majority of ombudsman advisory board members and long-term staff in New York City agree that voluntary community organizations should have the responsibility for administering the local long-term care ombudsman program. Eighty-seven percent of advisory and 71.4 percent of institutional representative respondents in the New York City study were of this opinion. The chief advantages of voluntary program auspices were seen to be their objectivity and independence. The belief was also expressed that the voluntary organization, in the case of the New York City program, has proved that it can adequately perform such a function and that it is more likely to be caring and concerned than public sponsors.

In the minority of cases where a division of government was preferred as the proper administrative location, the reasons given referred to these public entities as having a greater measure of authority and resources.

The Supervisory Function

Each volunteer ombudsman is accountable to a supervisor. Supervisory meetings are held at least once a month within the assigned facility or by telephone. When supervision is conducted in the field, the ombudsman is usually accompanied on rounds in order that an evaluation of performance may be carried out. Ombudsmen are also able to telephone their supervisor and discuss two aspects of a complaint: its substance or a strategy for resolution. Conferences with the ombudsmen and review of their contact register sheets enable the supervisor to ascertain the status of volunteer activities in each facility.

When asked about the desirability of additional supervisory help that might be offered by ombudsman program staff in the future, 72 percent of volunteer ombudsmen singled out the need to learn additional grievance resolution skills and techniques. A second cluster of needed supervisory help tended to emphasize the perceived need for peer and individual support as well as alternative methods for bolstering their technical skills, such as more opportunities to attend workshops and conferences on long-term care and to receive materials on understanding the aged. Least needed were materials on advocacy and alterations in the intensity or frequency of supervisory contacts in the field.

Among those volunteers who responded to inquiries concerning how ombudsman program staff could be most helpful to them, the majority stressed the importance of personal support and "pep talks" to neutralize the stress of the assignment. They also emphasized the benefit to be derived from the receipt of technical guidance. Volunteers maintained that they most often sought supervisory assistance for patients' rights and health care complaint cases whereas they were more likely to turn directly to nursing home administrators when dealing with administrative grievances.

Training

All volunteers participate in an initial six-day training session operated in conjunction with the New York State Office for the Aging and with the participation of other professionals in the field of long-term care. Training topics have encompassed:

1. Descriptions of the institutionalized aged propulation
2. Long-term care facility structure and level of care
3. Entitlements and benefits
4. Problem identifiction, investigation, and resolution procedures
5. Interviewing skills
6. Attitudinal, physiological, and psychological aspects of aging.

This phase of training is followed by monthly in-service training meetings with fellow ombudsmen at which time speakers from regulatory agencies and long-term care facilities are invited to speak and problems experienced in the facility are discussed.

Ombudsmen were asked to identify in descending order the three most helpful aspects of these training sessions, and similarly the three aspects of work for which the sessions did not prepare them very well. The training component viewed as most helpful was information received on the process of aging and institutionalization. Of less but nevertheless considerable value was information on complaint processing procedures and information on nursing home operations. Material pertaining to the external ombudsman program support network and training methods generally (role-playing) were deemed of least benefit. Findings suggest that even though information on aging, institutionalization, nursing home procedures, and complaint processing was quite helpful when presented, the volunteers nevertheless did not feel fully prepared to address these complex aspects of long-term care ombudsmanship, once they were actually assigned to a facility.

Ombudsman Facility Interaction

An outline of the "ideal type" of ombudsman/facility interaction process is presented here, as extracted from the New York City nursing home patient ombudsman program (NHPOP) training materials.[22]

I. *Introduction of Program to New Facility*
  A. NHPOP sends letter and brochure to facility requesting meeting.
  B. Program director and/or appropriate field staff meet with administrator to discuss placement of ombudsmen in the facility.
      1. Administrator and the NHPOP agree upon verification and problem-resolution process, as well as the designation of appropriate facility staff to work with ombudsmen.
      2. Program and facility staff agree as to the specific assignments for ombudsmen. The usual ratio is one ombudsman to 80–100 residents.
II. *Preparation of Facility for Program*
  A. Administrator informs staff about the program. NHPOP staff are available to explain the program at staff meetings, in-service training sessions, family and residents' council meetings.
  B. Administrator arranges the necessary introductions to ensure cooperation and plans for:
      1. Introduction of ombudsmen to facility

    2. Access to department heads and charge nurses for verification of complaints

    3. Half-hour weekly meetings between ombudsmen and staff designated to resolve verified problem/complaints

    4. Regular meetings with field supervisor to discuss unresolved and/or recurring problems

III. *Orientation of Ombudsmen to the Facility*

  A. Field supervisor and ombudsmen meet with available department heads for half an hour on first day of entry into facility. Discussion includes explanation of the program and special features of that particular facility.

  B. New ombudsmen tour facility and are introduced to staff on assigned floors. This usually takes an hour.

IV. *Program's Activities in the Facility*

  A. Ombudsmen

    1. Visits assigned floors for four to six hours each week.

    2. Verify identified problems/complaints with appropriate nursing home staff, usually charge nurse or department head.

    3. Meet as necessary with staff person assigned to resolve problems/complaints identified and verified by the ombudsmen. Confidentiality is respected, and the identity of residents is disclosed only with their permission.

  B. *Interaction Between NHPOP Staff and Facility Staff*

    1. Field supervisor is available to talk with facility staff should there be any problems with ombudsmen's activities.

    2. Field supervisor meets periodically with administrator or designated staff person to discuss any problems which may be unresolved at ombudsman/facility staff level.

    3. NHPOP shares monthly data reports with facility.

    4. Program director is available for consultation.

This outline represents the program's operational mode. The extent to which day-to-day activities conform to that normative framework will be examined in the following section.

Patient/Ombudsman Interactions

Data on the interactions between volunteer ombudsmen and residents have repeatedly emphasized the importance of individualized approaches to service delivery. Volunteers described the process of establishing communication with the institutionalized aged with the following phrases: "being friendly and unaggressive"; "being cheerful"; "sitting, touching, listening"; "having a friendly, personal attitude"; "establishing trust and finding common ground for communication"; "being a good listener and friend," and so forth. In the case of withdrawn patients, gradual introductions, nonverbal forms of communication, and confidence-building were stressed as well as the importance of repetitive, regularized contacts without imposing one's presence. Building trust and forming friendships were key elements throughout. This type of approach coupled with assurances of confidentiality remained the primary strategy that was used even when ombudsmen had to deal with the fear of staff reprisal, repeatedly mentioned by residents who lodged complaints.

Examples from the Florida program illustrate the varying degrees of case complexity that ombudsmen contend with daily:

The daughter of a nursing home resident complained that her mother's bracelet and wedding ring had disappeared two months earlier. The matter had been reported to the administrator but was not resolved. Then the mother's dresses began to disappear. The complainant reported to some of the home's staff that she had seen another resident wearing one of the dresses. The staff indicated nothing could be done about retrieving the mother's personal property.

A patient had been at a nursing home for three years as a private pay patient and then had to rely on Medicaid. Shortly thereafter the patient was transferred to a hospital on the basis of possible pneumonia. After two days' observation, the hospital could not confirm the home's diagnosis. The patient's relative called to complain that, on release from the hospital on the third day, the nursing home indicated that the patient could not return due to a lack of available beds.

A woman complained that her mother was restrained in a wheelchair by a bed sheet and not released for several hours, thus requiring the mother to sit in a puddle of urine. The complainant added that the nursing home did not have a physician's order requesting such restraint.

An elderly resident wandered away from a nursing home on Thanksgiving Day. She was found dead from exposure four days later in a wooded area about one mile from the facility. Police related that they had previously received numerous reports of residents wandering from this facility.[23]

Facility Staff/Ombudsman Interactions

Having gained access to the facility, volunteer ombudsmen can be expected to have different degrees of contact with various departments and individuals. Volunteers indicated that directors of social services were most often approached in this regard followed by directors of nursing and the facility administrators.

Ombudsman program literature stresses that the duties of the volunteer should not include provision of personal care (feeding and toileting), personal assistance (shopping, writing letters), or reading of medical charts. While institutional representatives were in general agreement that these were not appropriate ombudsmen tasks, they warned about two additional practices that ought to be avoided—the monitoring of staff practices and concern with medical treatment. Facility staff were more likely to emphasize the inappropriateness of these activities than the volunteer's participation in aspects of personal care or access to patients' records. Furthermore, approximately one in every three long-term care staff members believed that ombudsmen had actually entered into a "forbidden" territory that was beyond their competence and jurisdiction, and ignored the established procedures in performing their tasks. Administrators thus felt that volunteers had wrongfully attempted to become involved with patients' records or the monitoring of facility staff. On the other hand, directors of nursing described cases involving issues of medical care and treatment and social service directors emphasized that the volunteer had overstepped into the area of personal assistance.

After negotiating their entrance to a nursing home facility, ombudsmen make their preliminary exchanges with the facility's staff and also become acquainted with the residents. It does not take long before misunderstandings erupt concerning what the ombudsman is permitted to do. The three main staff groups—administrators, nurses, and social service personnel—usually try to prevent these external agents from stepping into their traditional domains. Tensions linger, and conflicts remain unresolved. Ombudsman program staff, meanwhile, realize they must marshal external supports if they wish to achieve a modicum of effectiveness.

Interorganizational Relations

The next logical step in this inquiry was to determine the extent of program involvement with external organizations, both at the public and the voluntary level, and to assess their contributions to the development of an ombudsman presence in long-term care institutions. In order to tap the types of organizational endeavors through which external associations become involved with nursing home ombudsman programs, a scale of participatory activities was constructed for the national survey and found internally reliable. State ombudsman respondents were asked to indicate on a four-point scale how often citizens' organizations engage in a variety of participatory activities with the ombudsman program. Citizens' organizations were said to be maximally engaged in the most passive of the activities listed, namely, the dissemination of ombudsman program information. While this is an important activity, it seemingly provides the least amount of opportunity for mutual involvement in the planning and execution of ombudsman services for the aged. Joint lobbying and the forming of a long-term care network with the program were ranked second in frequency.

Increasingly independent activities, such as offering community consumer education, volunteer pools, and the monitoring of the ombudsman program by voluntary citizens' organizations, were cited as occurring with only medium frequency. Highly independent citizens' group activity, such as the actual sponsoring of an ombudsman program, the training of ombudsman volunteers, and active opposition to the ombudsman program, were found by state ombudsmen to be the least frequent among the activities rated.

In the course of the observational field visits, researchers noticed instances in which citizens' organizations were actively involved in the planning and execution of ombudsman services for the institutionalized elderly. The Oregon nursing home ombudsman maintained ongoing activities with an umbrella organization of thirty-eight senior organizations called United Seniors, and with the Gray Panthers. The Minnesota nursing home ombudsman program worked very closely with the Minnesota Senior Federation and local advocacy and resident's council organizations. The Michigan program was actually sponsored by an independent citizens' advocacy organization, CBC. Such affiliations, it seems, are the exception rather than the rule in the majority of the states.

Relations with citizens' organizations were viewed in the larger framework of interorganizational contacts that ombudsman programs also maintain. State nursing home ombudsmen were asked to rank on a scale of one to five the frequency and perceived value of contacts with a range of eleven organizations in the long-term care network. Organizations with which the state ombudsmen maintained the most frequent contact were governmental service and regulatory agencies: state offices on aging, state health departments, and state public welfare departments, with some minor internal switching of respective rank.

The grouping that provided the second most frequent stream of contacts was that of the activist organizations: legal services developers, state voluntary advocacy organizations, and local grass-roots advocacy groups. Once again, with some internal reordering, this group as a whole was found to offer the second most beneficial set of contacts. Finally, the last group constituting organizations with the least frequent contact with the ombudsman program included the associations of proprietary long-term care facilities, legislative committees, associations of not-for-profit long-term care facilities, and the governor's office. This group of long-term care providers, legislators, and chief executives also resulted in the least beneficial of all the organizational contacts undertaken by the ombudsman program.

The question must be raised, therefore, whether the frequency of contacts causes a raised perception as to the benefit of those contacts or, vice versa, whether unfruitful contacts lead to a decrease in their frequency. In any event, the complexity of interorganizational relations necessarily requires that nursing home ombudsmen devote a considerable amount of time and effort to public relations management with representatives of the service bureaucracy, long-term care providers, public officials, and citizens' organizations.

An important organizational link that was not tapped by the survey instrument but whose significance became apparent as a result of the on-site interviews was the relationship between the ombudsman program and the local Area Agency of Aging (AAAs). The Triple As are often seen as major obstacles to the effective implementation of long-term care ombudsman services. This is indeed ironic in that the AAAs were established to develop a community-based focus for the planning and delivery of services for the aged.

The reason for the lack of rapport between the ombudsman program and the AAA, according to the former, is that AAAs primarily contract with providers for the delivery of concrete, direct services (meals, transportation, counseling, home care). Local ombudsman services diverge from this pattern in three significant ways: (1) they are a mediation service as opposed to a traditional direct service; (2) they are often attached to an AAA administratively, therefore requiring supervision as well as fiscal support; and (3) they focus on institutional settings which have not been the traditional target of the Older Americans Act mandate. Finally, AAAs are said to be resistant to providing additional resources beyond those which the Older Americans Act requires in support of ombudsman programming (one percent of the Title III-B funds for social services or $20,000, whichever is higher). Many AAAs, it is believed, would prefer to see even this base-line support earmarked for the purchase of concrete community services as compared to the provision of mediation services for the aged in institutions.

Conclusion

State ombudsman programs differ in terms of administrative location, centralization of function, statutory empowerment, patterns of staffing, professional/volunteer ratio, scope of serviced populations and primary program focus, be it on licensure, patients' rights, or interactional issues. Despite their obvious heterogeneity, unmistakable patterns of working strategies have taken shape. Some evolved into model approaches later on, to be adopted by the more recently constituted state programs. Five such prototypes, placed at different points along a collaborative-contest continuum and in terms of tasks allocation between state and local levels of operation, were reviewed in detail.

Gaining access to local facilities and establishing communication with both staff and residents is the initial evidence that local ombudsman programs have gotten off the ground. Interactions between ombudsmen and facilities are, however, a complex process that requires careful systematization if the intent is to ensure a relatively smooth operation. It includes the definition of roles and mutual expectations, as well as the sequencing of steps in the grievance resolution process. Tensions inevitably erupt between the "insiders," the facilities staff, and the external agents, the ombudsmen. The latter seek to bolster their precarious status by harnessing support from the community at large—and here lies their dilemma: the more effort they invest in public relations management, the fewer resources are left for attending to their primary advocacy function.

CHAPTER FIVE
What Do Ombudsmen Do?

This chapter presents findings on the roles that nursing home ombudsmen perform and the extent to which the corresponding role prescriptions are accepted by long-term care staff and the institutionalized aged. How the ombudsman's role is perceived and the extent to which it is legitimized in the institutional setting merit primary consideration here.

Three broad categories of possible ombudsman function have been derived from the literature on interventive behavior (see chapter 1). Programs may first align themselves with the "classical" notion of an impartial mediator who is functionally independent, nonjudgmental, and nonpartisan. Such ombudsmen, while capable at times of some hard bargaining between administration and citizen, tend more usually to associate themselves with the original Swedish conceptualization of the rather detached arbitrator.

A second approach moves toward a greater identification with political or partisan stances. In such cases, the ombudsman may approximate the role of an advocate engaging in open confrontations and taking sides with a particular party in the dispute. This role, in contrast to the classical stance, clearly tends to be a more active one, reflecting a results-oriented perspective.

Finally, a third functional orientation, a hybrid type, may be labeled as the "therapeutically supportive" ombudsman. This individual focuses on the provision of emotional support and the expression of friendly concern or caring. The effort here is to prevent the weaker party from suffering unnecessary psychological pain or discomfort in its interactions with a dominant authority.

Whatever the orientation followed, the ombudsman's objective is to improve the quality of life of the citizen, or in the case of long-term care, the resident/patient. Each of these three orientations tends to pursue its objective through different service strategies, and yet their role dimensions are not entirely self-contained or mutually exclusive.

Each perspective includes, indeed, a range of possible behaviors, and each may partially overlap with the other. Felton et al. sought precisely to merge the functions of the patient advocate, integrator and therapist, the result being a new kind of professional, the "mental health generalist."[1] Mailick's study of patient-representative programs in short-term general hospitals suggested that such services may have overlapping functions but that one can distinguish among four types: a complaint processor, a personal service (counseling), a financial service, and a hospitality/personal courtesy role.[2] Regan, in turn, strongly argued for a combination of patients' advocate and impartial mediator tasks.[3]

In an initial assessment of the first nursing home ombudsman demonstrations in the United States, the AoA's nursing home interests staff recommended no less than ten different roles or functions that nursing home ombudsmen should fulfill, including both partisan and nonpartisan stances.[4] Forman's analysis of these same programs reemphasized the varied application of the ombudsman concept and a multiplicity of roles with which programs may identify.[5] Linnane similarly pointed out that the ombudsman must choose a role which best fits the nature of the complaint, including those of broker, mediator, educator, planner, and advocate.[6]

Research Procedures

A series of program perception measures was constructed and tested during the study to assess the nature of intra- and intergroup views of ombudsman roles and functions. Respondents were questioned as to the accuracy of a series of eleven potential role behaviors in characterizing the activities of the nursing home patient ombudsman. The role behaviors in reference constituting the role perception scale were:

1. Making easier the conditions of residents
2. Guiding the resident through the proper channels
3. Serving as a middleman between the nursing home and the resident
4. Arguing the cause of the resident
5. Serving as an impartial listener
6. Translating the rules and regulations of nursing home residents
7. Explaining decisions of others to residents
8. Observing staff practices in nursing homes
9. Reforming and improving staff practices in nursing homes
10. Occupying a watchdogging position to insure adequate nursing home conditions
11. Providing emotional support to residents/patients.

The five-point metric scale of accuracy ranged from very accurate to not accurate at all. Respondents were then asked to identify in descending order, the three most important role behaviors for ombudsmen in nursing homes, thus providing data on perceptions of "actual" and "desired" program functions.

Composite measures of individual perceptions along three hypothesized behavioral role dimensions (I = mediator; II = advocate; and III = therapeutic supporter) were derived by means of the judgments of a ten-member expert panel. The panel, composed of academicians and service practitioners throughout New York State and Connecticut with acknowledged expertise in the field of social welfare, was asked to judge the "degree of fit" of the original series of eleven role behaviors within the three broader behavioral dimensions. Utilization of the Student-Neuman-Keuls procedure to identify ranges for the less than .05 level enabled the researchers to assign seven of the eleven original role behavior items to the three behavioral dimensions. Table 5.1 identifies the internal scale items validated for inclusion within each of the three behavioral dimensions of program function. Also presented in the table are the results of reliability analysis for each dimension obtained in the first study (New York City). As measures of internal consistency, the Cronbach standardized item alphas obtained (ranging from .65 to .88) are quite acceptable when one considers the limited number of scale items within each composite measure. The standardized item alpha obtained for the same role perception scale in the national study was .91. Internal correlation coefficients between all role items ranged from .12 to .61 in the New York study and from .20 to .76 in the national project.

Table 5.1
Scale Item Information and Reliability Analysis (Standardized Item Alphas) for Composite Program Perception Measures (New York City Study)

Program Perception Measure	Number of Scale Items	Identity of Scale Items	Standardized Item Alpha (α) (Internal Consistency)
Role behavior scale	11	Role 1–Role 11	.88
Mediator role scale	2	Role 3 = middleman	
		Role 7 = explainer	.65
Advocate role scale	3	Role 4 = arguer	
		Role 9 = reformer	
		Role 10 = watchdog	.69
Therapeutic support scale	2	Role 1 = easer of conditions	
		Role 11 = provider of emotional support	.67

Perceived Role Behaviors

National Perspective

As spelled out in the section on methodology (chapter 3), the national long-term care network queried in this study was composed of representatives from the following groups: (1)

state commissioners and directors on aging; (2) legal services
developers from advocacy assistance units; (3) state commissioners of health; (4) state commissioners of welfare; (5) state-
level, not-for-profit nursing home associations; (6) proprietary
nursing home associations; and (7) citizens' advocacy organizations. Trends identified in the data revealed that the network, for the sake of comparison, could be disaggregated into
three affinal subgroups reflecting similar response perspectives across a range of questions:

1. *Aging interest group.* Comprised of the commissioners on aging,
   legal services developers, and citizens' organizations
2. *Human service commissioners.* Including the health and welfare
   commissioners
3. *Long-term care providers.* Combining both not-for-profit and proprietary nursing home organizations.

Where appropriate, the responses of the state nursing home
ombudsmen have been included in the aging interest group
as well.

It became initially apparent that the three major respondent
groups do not agree in their definition of ombudsman role
behaviors. Significant differences were found, in fact, on the
relative perception of role accuracy. All eleven of the role-de-
scription items developed in the New York City study showed
significant variation across the three major national groups defined earlier. Furthermore, except for the two roles rated least
accurate by the aging interest group—the reformer and
watchdog roles—even the lowest of the remaining nine roles
was still higher in absolute score than the most accurate score
assigned to all role descriptions by human services commissioners and by long-term care providers. The latter respondent groups were less willing than the aging interest group to
grant conclusive or unequivocal ratings to almost any ombudsman activity, a fact that may be interpreted as resistance toward legitimatizing the functions and boundaries of the om-

budsman role and/or ignorance as to how the local ombudsman mandate is being carried out.

Viewing each role item separately, a consistent pattern becomes apparent: each role is rated most accurately by the aging interest group, second most accurately by the human services comissioners, and least accurately by the long-term care providers. When group rating values are considered, it can be seen that the aging interest group viewed all but the reformer and watchdog role descriptions as highly accurate. The human service commissioners granted a less conclusive degree of accuracy to the same group of roles while the long-term care providers were largely indifferent to the degree of correctness reflected by each role description.

Some variations are also discernible in the internal relative rankings of the accuracy of the roles by each major respondent groups. "Arguing the cause of the resident" was accepted as the most accurate role description by the human services commissioners but one of the least accurate by the aging interest group. The differences in this case may stem more from varying semantic interpretations than from actual role differences. The aging interest group, in turn, viewed the translation of regulations for residents as a highly accurate role, a perception not shared by human services commissioners or by long-term care providers. Human services commissioners, on the other hand, saw watchdogging as relatively more accurate among the list of roles than did the aging interest group. Finally, the long-term care providers assigned relatively high accuracy to the provision of emotional support, a role viewed as less accurate by the other two respondent groups.

These last differences primarily reflect internal ranking disparities between groups. The major finding remains the presence of significant difference in the perceptions of ombudsman behavior across the major groups, and particularly the reluctance of the long-term care providers to legitimize any role as a proper portrait of local ombudsman activity.

New York City Perspective

New York City respondents included a different set of population categories than the national sample. The volunteer ombudsmen and their local advisory board members were subsumed in a category labeled "external agents." The administrative directors of participating nursing homes, in combination with their nursing and social service directors, constitute in turn the polar category of internal agents or representatives. Both groups coincided in according higher accuracy to the therapeutic cluster of roles and lesser accuracy to the advocate one. The mediator role, most closely associated with the classical definition of ombudsman, lies between.

While the relative positioning of each behavioral dimension is identical for each group, the extent of difference between totals, according to an analysis of variance, indicates that the degree of accuracy assigned to each behavioral cluster differs significantly among the groups. This difference is so great, in fact, that the least accurate behavioral dimension in the opinion of all external agents (ombudsman as advocate) is accorded higher accuracy than the most accurate dimension in the opinion of long-term care staff (ombudsman as therapist). It would appear that persons directly associated with the operation of the program have a more clear and definitive sense of what the ombudsman role is all about. Long-term care staff, on the other hand, have a more distorted notion of what the ombudsmen are actually doing in their own facilities. Their assignment of less accurate scores to each of the three potential role dimensions suggests a resistance or lack of clarity about the purpose of the volunteers' efforts. It should be remembered that this trend is identical to that which appeared in the national study.

It is worth noting here that both subgroups of external program agents—the ombudsmen volunteers and their advisory board members—tend to be in close ideological agreement regarding the activities of the volunteers even though current program structure does not allow sustained contact between them. Intragroup agreement tends to hold for all three groups of internal agents or long-term care staff as well, though nursing home administrators, who have less contact with ombudsman than any other staff population, tend to diverge in the direction of role blurring.

In order to determine the degree of differential accuracy accorded to each of the three behavioral clusters within each respondent population, tests of significance were performed between pairs of actual program dimensions. As expected, both volunteer ombudsmen and their advisory board members are in close accord. Taken together, they consider the therapeutic role to be significantly more reflective of actual ombudsman activities than either the advocate or the mediator roles. At the same time, the mediator role is seen to be a measurably more accurate descriptor for the volunteers' efforts than that of an advocate.

Taken together, long-term care staff largely concur in assigning the advocate role significantly less accuracy than the mediator or the therapeutic role. However, long-term care staff do not differentiate between mediative efforts and the provision of therapeutic support. The perceptions of long-term care staff seem to waver between the two, thus confirming their uncertainty on the issue.

Attitudes Toward the Ombudsman Role

This section reveals the feelings of long-term care staff as to whether the role of ombudsman is necessary, or whether it constitutes an invasion into their own professional domain. Respondents in the New York City study were asked whether ombudsmen should be placed in all nursing homes, and whether they duplicate the work of the patients' advocate, of the New York State Department of Health. They were also questioned as to whether most problems the ombudsmen deal with would be eventually resolved by the nursing home staff. Moreover, is there a tendency for ombudsmen to inflate artificially the number of complaints by encouraging patients' griping? Do ombudsmen constitute an unwelcomed burden on the facilities? And finally, are they adequately trained for this role?

The three groups of long-term care staff—nursing home administrators, directors of social services, and directors of nursing—were in agreement that ombudsman programs should be found in all long-term care facilities, but at the same time they mildly agreed that the types of problems brought to the ombudsmen would eventually be resolved by nursing home staff anyway if an ombudsman were not there. Nursing home administrators were most convinced of this.

Staff did not believe that the ombudsman duplicates the work of the New York State Department of Health Office of the Patient Advocate (an office that responds to reports of abused patients and has recognized statutory and regulatory authority), though, again, administrators were less convinced than departmental directors. Similarly, staff generally did not perceive the ombudsman to be a governmental "regulator" or investigator. Staff were in close agreement in their belief that the ombudsman is not likely to promote complaining and griping by residents. They believed even more strongly that the program does not create another burden on the facility, although there is significant variance concerning the extent to which this is the case: social service directors were more convinced that the ombudsman program is "burdensome" (it is possible that directors of social service saw the ombudsmen more likely to tread on their professional turf due to conceivable overlap in their roles). Finally, staff was uniformly convinced that ombudsmen do not receive enough preparation and training to perform their jobs adequately. They felt that the volunteers have only been "fairly" to "not very well" equipped to perform their jobs. The reason most often given to explain this deficiency was poor training. Less often mentioned was the volunteers' lack of previous experience and concern.

Statistically significant correlations were found between staff belief that the program should be found in all long-term care facilities and their belief that it fills a service gap, is effective, has impact, and should be high in priority. On the other hand, as they express greater certainty that ombudsmen lack training, they are also more likely to perceive the program as filling less of a service gap, being less effective, less impacting and of lower priority.

What emerges from these data is the absence of strongly negative or antagonistic reactions to the ombudsman concept but rather the belief that more training and preparation of volunteers are necessary before the idea can be successfully put into operation. Those staff groups that expressed normative acceptance of the concept and role were more likely to perceive the program's efforts as successful. Those convinced of inadequacies in training held more negative views of program performance altogether.

At no point did any long-term care staff groups notice negative reactions by other individuals to the ombudsman program. Perceived in-house responses range from mildly positive to relative indifference. It is noteworthy that as a group, long-term care staff believed that social service staff, administrative personnel, and patients have reacted most positively to the volunteers. Furthermore, in five out of six cases it was the social service directors who perceived the reactions of facility groups to be less positive than their administrative and nursing counterparts. In one case—the perceived reaction of professional nurses—this difference of opinion was strongly significant, while in a second case—the perceived reactions of nonprofessional staff—intergroup variance bordered on being significant. When asked to provide the reasons for various in-house responses to the volunteers' presence, the belief that the latter represented potential sources of constructive criticism and were nonthreatening was voiced considerably more often than the reverse.

Desired Role Behaviors

National Study

Interviewees in the national study were asked to indicate the three most important roles that the nursing home ombudsman should play. The roles were selected from the list of behavioral descriptions included in the role perception scale. Respondents were also asked to indicate the three most important issues that the nursing home ombudsman program should address. The data collected in these two instances reflected the respondents' preferences on two key aspects of this long-term care quality assurance program: which area should merit the attention of the ombudsman and how that attention should be expressed.

The data were submitted to factor analysis in order to identify study group orientations. Responses were prepared by assigning them weighted scores prior to the factorial procedure. The most important choice received a score of four, the second most important choice a score of two, and the third most important choice a score of one. The remainder of the items were considered to have a score of zero. The raw data were then subjected to the principal component method of factor analysis. The factors were rotated by varimax method to a final position. Individual scores were generated for each respondent on each derived factor. Group mean factor scores were then computed for each of the eight original respondent groups.

A review of the final factor solutions shows that the first factor exhibited high positive loading on the consensual, collaborative roles of guiding the resident through the proper channels, acting as middleman and as impartial listener. High negative loadings, on the other hand, were obtained for reformer and watchdog roles, and arguing the cause of the resident. This factor may, therefore, be said to reflect a continuum that spans from collaborative to contest-oriented role perceptions.

The second factor revealed a high negative loading on the middleman role, and high positive loadings on impartial listening, providing emotional support, and easing conditions. The continuum of role choices represented in this factor, therefore, may be characterized as one that ranges from broker to therapist perceptions. The visual representation of plotted group mean scores, appearing in Figure 5.1, is instructive.

It can be seen that the group most contest-oriented consists of the citizen organizations, followed closely by the legal services developers. Commissioners on aging and welfare were somewhat inclined toward assigning an adversary orientation to the ombudsman role. Furthest from the contest perception, and therefore reflecting a collaborative orientation, were the two long-term care provider associations. The providers were followed by commissioners of health and state ombudsmen, the latter of whom were relatively less consensually bound than the other "collaboratively oriented" groups.

Viewing the broker/therapist continuum, it is obvious that the long-term care providers identified most directly with the therapeutic version of the ombudsman role, closely followed by the commissioners of welfare. All the remaining groups preferred the middleman role, with the ombudsmen themselves expressing the most preference for this nonconfrontational, nonpartisan stance. Considering each group's placement along the two role choice dimensions, it can be seen that notable distinctions occur.

The not-for-profit and proprietary nursing home associations clearly showed preference for a contest-free ombudsman role which focuses solely upon the provision of emotional support to the nursing home patient. The aging interest group (the commissioners of aging, legal services developers, and citizens' advocacy organizations) preferred the opposite role composition: a contest-oriented ombudsman who actively intercedes for residents in nursing facilities. The human services commissioners were divided on the question, with commissioners of welfare therapeutically oriented but with a subsidiary contest bent and the commissioners of health collaboratively inclined toward the brokerage role. The state

Figure 5.1
Role Choices for Nursing Home Ombudsmen

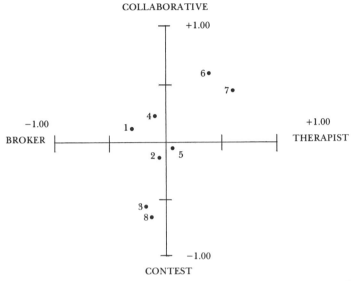

1 = state ombudsmen 2 = commissioners on aging 3 = legal services 4 = commissioners of health 5 = commissioners of welfare 6 = not-for-profit associations 7 = proprietary associations 8 = citizens' organizations

Key to Figure 5.1

		GROUP MEAN FACTOR SCORES	
		Collaborative/ Contest	Broker/ Therapist
GROUP	*FREQUENCY*	*FACTOR*	*FACTOR*
1. State ombudsmen	42	0.15	−0.28
2. Commissioners on aging	42	−0.15	−0.05
3. Legal services	34	−0.56	−0.17
4. Commissioner of health	34	0.25	−0.10
5. Commissioner of welfare	28	−0.02	0.02
6. Not-for-profit associations	26	0.59	0.39
7. Proprietary associations	29	0.47	0.58
8. Citizens' organizations	30	−0.59	−0.15

ombudsmen themselves favored the mediative broker role, but with emphasis on a collaborative orientation.

The same type of analysis was made for the second set of items in regard to preferred program directions. The issues included were:

1. Residents' rights
2. Abuse of residents
3. Nursing home regulations/enforcement
4. Medicaid discrimination
5. Upgrading nursing home staff
6. Relocation trauma
7. Boarding home standards (adult homes, residential care facilities

8. Consumer education relating to long-term care
9. Alternatives to institutionalization in long-term care
10. Mental health needs of long-term care facility residents
11. Abuse of residents' funds
12. Residents participation in facility governance

The results were equally, if not more, definitive than in the preceding analysis. The first factor had high negative loadings on issues of abuse of residents and residents' rights, and high positive loadings on alternatives to institutionalization, community consumer education, and mental health needs of long-term care residents. This factor may be characterized, therefore, as one that spans a continuum from rights-oriented, watchdog issues to developmental, personal growth issues.

The second factor had high positive loadings on the issue of boarding home standards and high negative loadings on consumer education and resident participation in facility governance. The range of issues that are reflected in this continuum may thus be considered to extend from a facility orientation to a resident/consumer focus. The configuration of group responses is visually presented in Figure 5.2.

The plot of each group's preferred issue focus for the ombudsman program underscores the division of the respondents into three major clusters. The long-term care provider groups were distinguishable from the remainder of the respondents in their preference for a developmental issue focus. The remainder of the study groups preferred the watchdog focus. At the same time, the human services commissioners were distinguishable from the aging interest group in their preference for a more resident/consumer focus. The latter indicated a preference for a facility focus to their watchdogging efforts.

Figure 5.2
Issue Focus for Nursing Home Ombudsmen

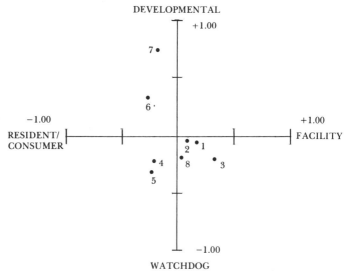

1 = state ombudsmen 2 = commissioners on aging 3 = legal services 4 = commissioners of health 5 = commissioners of welfare 6 = not-for-profit associations 7 = proprietary associations 8 = citizens' organizations

Key to Figure 5.2

		GROUP MEAN FACTOR SCORES	
		Developmental/ Watchdog	Resident/ Facility
GROUP	*FREQUENCY*	*FACTOR*	*FACTOR*
1. State ombudsmen	42	−0.05	0.21
2. Commissioners on aging	42	−0.01	0.07
3. Legal services	34	−0.20	0.32
4. Commissioners of health	34	−0.21	−0.19
5. Commissioners of welfare	28	−0.34	−0.22
6. Not-for-profit associations	26	0.38	−0.26
7. Proprietary associations	29	0.75	−0.17
8. Citizens' organizations	30	−0.18	0.04

In essence, the aging interest group (state ombudsmen included) reiterated in this national survey their inclination toward an ombudsman program that focuses on watchdogging facility issues. The long-term care provider group underscored an opposing orientation as they emphasized the need to target on the individual resident or consumer needs and staying away from the institutional facility. The human services commissioner group wavered between these two positions. They tend toward the watchdogging orientation but with a focus upon the residents' rights rather than on the long-term care facility itself.

New York Study

A first analysis of the New York City data shows no significant difference between nursing home staff and the external agents (ombudsmen and community advisory board members) concerning desired role behaviors. Closer inspection does, however, suggest more subtle differences within the respondent groups. Again the advocate/contest role is given lowest priority by all respondents. Furthermore, external agents no longer differentiate between behavioral dimensions with the certainty they possessed when assessing the accuracy of actual ombudsman roles. Thus, while the therapeutic role is still ranked highest, it achieves a lower level of significant difference in relation to the advocate function than earlier. In addition, the therapeutic stance is no longer considered significantly more important than the mediator role nor is the mediator role ranked higher than the advocate role.

Analysis of long-term care staff data shows congruence between their perceptions of actual and desired role identity for ombudsmen, suggesting more consistency between the normative and experiential levels. Long-term care employees are perhaps perceiving ombusmen as doing those things that they would want or expect the ombudsman to do. Staff respondents thus continue to maintain that mediative and therapeutic functions are more critical modes of ombudsman intervention than the advocative or partisan stance.

It is worth mentioning that nursing directors assign greatest importance to mediative strategies, whereas social service directors consider the therapeutic mode as the primary one.

Again, administrators waver between these two behavioral clusters. In any case, staff findings taken together suggest that mediative and therapeutic support roles tend to be compounded and overlap, whereas the ombudsmen and their community advisors keep them apart, suggesting a more complex or pluralistic view. This would include classical, nonpartisan, and confrontational approaches, depending on the particular needs of the aged resident.

Volunteer ombudsmen and facilities staff in New York City were asked to assess the importance of dominant personality traits in determining program effectiveness. Seven such traits were listed in the research questionnaire: "caring, warm"; "optimistic, enthusiastic"; "aggressive"; "patient, perseverant"; "intelligent"; "diplomatic, objective"; and "tough." The relative importance given to these various behavioral traits is consistent with the preceding data concerning desired role behaviors. Caring, warmth, and solicitous concern, all therapeutic characteristics, were assigned greatest priority by the volunteer ombudsmen, followed by the need to act with diplomatic tact and objective detachment, obviously mediative traits. Least often mentioned was the need to be tough—in fact, it was never mentioned—followed by aggressive confrontational qualities, an allusion to the advocate role.

Long-term care staff assigned equal, and even the greatest, weight to the "capacity to be caring/warm" and "diplomatic/objective." Conversely, they gave lower priority to the attributes of toughness, perseverance, and aggressiveness. Interestingly, all respondent groups placed relatively little import on such qualities as intelligence or good judgment. Does it suggest that these are not necessarily relevant to showing care and concern or to being diplomatic within the nursing home setting? Does it also imply that rational, instrumental activities are the staffs' exclusive province, while ombudsmen, like volunteer friendly visitors, should confine themselves to expressive conflict-free social pleasantries?

Nursing Home Residents Perception of Ombudsmen

While elderly residents were not required in the New York study to assess ombudsman functions, several questions yielded clues as to their views. To begin with, both ombudsmen and long-term care staff were in agreement that the institutionalized aged do not have a clear understanding of what ombudsmen are supposed to do and how to utilize this role to their benefit. Indeed, only 28.0 percent of the ombudsmen and 16.4 percent of the facility staff believed that patients have accurate perceptions of what the ombudsmen were doing in their homes. It is noteworthy that the nursing home administrators, as a group, were the most pessimistic concerning this issue with only 10.0 percent acknowledging that residents/patients are correct in their views of the ombudsman function.

When asked what expectations they thought the aged harbored with regard to ombudsmen, long-term care staff stressed that often residents simply did not know what to expect. In those cases where they believed that patients had recognizable expectations, they believed they centered on some combination of a personal support/friendly visitor and an advocate. They thought that the idea of an impartial mediator was alien to the residents' experience. Ombudsmen were similarly convinced that the aged were either ignorant on the matter or else apt to ascribe advocative and personalized characteristics to the ombudsman's interventive efforts. Ombudsmen concurred that the mediative function was one that the resident did not understand. Rather, they perceived that the older person probably identifies with partisan ombudsman stances whether they were of an aggressive political nature or a therapeutic bent.

When comparing long-term care staff and ombudsmen perceptions of residents' expectations with those of residents themselves, a high degree of consistency was obtained. Residents acknowledging awareness of the ombudsman program responded as to why they felt the continuation of the program was or was not important. Of those who felt it was important,

45 percent indicated that the volunteers served functions similar to those that might be expected of a friendly visitor ("She is nice to me and helpful"; "She asks me how I am," and so on), and 33 percent described more aggressive, advocacy-oriented functions ("They serve as inspectors"; she shows her "authority" and "power"; they "get results" and "make conditions better"; and so forth). The concept of a middleman or liaison between two parties remained conspicuously absent.

The State Ombudsman

Findings reported in this chapter relate for the most part to the local ombudsman, the volunteer front liner assigned to a specific facility or manageable number of nursing homes in the community. Consideration must also be given to the state ombudsman, a professional civil service position responsible for the planning, implementation, and overseeing of all ombudsman program activities within their state jurisdictions. The state ombudsman's role emanates from the nursing home ombudsman program which evolved over the last decade from at least three separate mandates. President Nixon's 1971 eight-point plan for improving nursing home care resulted in the first model ombudsman projects up until 1975. Subsequent program development funds were provided through AoA discretionary grants issued between 1975 and 1978 to any state desiring to implement a nursing home ombudsman program. Finally, the 1978 amendments to the Older American Act required all states to establish a long-term care ombudsman program. A quarter of the state ombudsman programs in the respondent sample were initiated during the model projects period, over half during the period of discretionary funding, and somewhat less than a fifth in the period from 1975 to the present when implementation of a long-term care ombudsman became mandated by federal law.

Few of the state ombudsmen active at the time of the survey dated their initial involvement to the early model projects days.

Rather, most traced their professional participation in any capacity in the program to the two latter periods. More reveal-
ing is the fact that about two thirds of the state nursing home
ombudsmen were appointed to the position of state ombudsman during the three years preceding the survey, while less
than a fifth of the same programs traced their beginnings to
that same period. The data thus strongly suggest that there
has been substantial turnover among the principal actors during the short life of this public program, and that no one individual had been witness to the evolution of long-term care
ombudsmanship efforts at the state level.

This fact is illustrated by the example of ombudsmen in the
field visit sample. Nine state ombusman programs had been
purposively chosen for observation due to their stability and
significant prototypical differences. Seven of the nine state
ombudsmen were actually veterans of the program, while two
were more recent appointees. Since the field visits in the summer of 1981, however, two of the nine ombudsmen interviewed have left their positions. This, combined with the survey data, reinforces the argument that staffing the central
administrative position in the state nursing home ombudsman
programmatic effort is characterized by a fair degree of inst-
ability. This matter will be discussed in chapter 7.

State nursing home ombudsmen came to their jobs with a
range of prior experience. While most had worked in the field
of aging generally, somewhat less than half had previously
worked in a nursing home or home for the aged. The vast
majority indicated prior experience with community-based social or health agencies. However, an equally vast majority indicated no experience in long-term care licensure or regulatory agencies. A profile is presented, therefore, of the nursing
home ombudsman as an individual experienced in aging and
human services, but less likely to have prior knowledge of the
long-term care facilitty or direct acquaintance with the rules
that regulate its function.

State ombudsmen were asked to rank the relative importance of six skills variously identified in the nursing home om-

budsman literature as necessary for the successful performance of the ombudsman role: complaint processing skills,
supportive counseling skills, legal activist skills, understanding
nursing home operations and procedures, sensitivity to the aging process and old people, and community organization skills.
In their responses, ombudsmen placed primary emphasis upon
the following three skills, in order of importance: (1) understanding nursing home operations; (2) sensitivity to the aging
process; and (3) complaint processing.

It is quite significant that they recognized as the area most
important to master the very one in which they indicated having the least experience. The skills of community organization
and supportive counseling were less highly ranked, perhaps
due to the respondents' stated experience in the human services. Finally, least emphasis was placed on legal activism, pos-
sibly underlining the ombudsmen's commitment to the role's
classical roots in impartiality and neutral mediation, as opposed to partisanship either in the former behavior of therapeutic support or aggressive advocacy. Thus it may be seen
that while the state nursing home ombudsmen do not necessarily come to the position with all the relevant prior experience, they do recognize the importance of, and the need to
obtain, such skills.

A view of the ways in which state ombudsmen perceive their
function, and the focus of the ombudsman program, is presented next. A range of respondent interpretations is indicated rather than a particular characteristic response regarding the program. Ombudsmen were asked to estimate on a
five-point scale the amount of time they devote to three dimensions of program activity: facilitating local ombudsman
program development, advocacy on behalf of individual complaints, and issue or system advocacy. Mean scores for all three
of the activity foci converge in the middle range, indicating
similar patterns of time allocation. While the individual complaint focus achieved a slightly lower time commitment rating,
statistical testing revealed the absence of significant difference
between it and the other activities. Therefore no single pro-

gram function was seen to represent the primary responsibility for state ombudsmen in long-term care.

The slightly reduced emphasis on individual complaints may reflect a process of natural program evolution. In its initial stages, the state-level ombudsman program necessarily acts in response to individual complaints in specific facilities. As the state program grows and matures, however, a characteristic development seems to be the transfer of responsibility for individual complaint resolution to local outposts of the ombudsman program. State nursing home ombudsman programs, in turn, accept increased responsibility for developing local ombudsman program capacity in the domain of individual advocacy at the same time that state programming in issues advocacy is expanding. Examples of this evolutionary process are seen in the Georgia long term care ombudsman program where state-level activity has shifted from complaint handling to support for area program development, through professional recruitment, training, and ongoing staff supervision. Similarly, the New York State nursing home program has targeted increased emphasis in such program capacity building in the western portion of the state, as has Michigan in its less densely populated areas. Both states have taken on regional ombudsmen in an effort to decentralize the handling of complaints.

Once a local capacity to act as nursing home ombudsman has been established, state-level programs turn to issue advocacy, using collected data on individual complaint handling as a primary source for issue identification. Thus the state ombudsman programs are turning more frequently to computerized management information systems to strengthen their capacity for addressing systemic long-term care issues. The Ohio State nursing home ombudsman program, for example, has developed a comprehensive computerized complaint reporting system. New York is currently experimenting with such a model. Other states' programs aspire to reach this level of technology.

The facilitation of local ombudsman program capacity is thus seen as a means by which state-level issues advocacy will be enhanced. How do the ombudsmen view their participation in the development of local programs' capacity? State ombudsmen respondents were asked to indicate the nature of their role vis-à-vis local program development: as a resource to provide technical assistance when so requested; as an equal partner with communities in developing programs and procedures; or as a leader with authority for the development of local programs.

While a plurality of state ombudsman respondents indicated the most directive or activistic of the suggested roles (as a leader with authority for local program development), no one role received a clear majority of responses. There is thus a variety of interpretations as to how the state-level ombudsman program intercedes on behalf of local program development. Again, it may be hypothesized that such variations may reflect different stages of the ombudsman program development process, as well as differing philosophies concerning the nature and goals of state ombudsman program efforts.

Complaints Handled by Ombudsmen

National Perspective

What are the most common complaints and problems brought to the ombudsman's attention? How amenable are they to proper resolution? State ombudsmen defined the most frequently addressed issues in the following order:

1. Residents' rights
2. Consumer education for long-term care
3. Nursing home regulation/enforcement
4. Abuse of residents
5. Alternatives to institutionalization.

All these, with the exception of nursing home regulation enforcement, were among the issues perceived as less difficult to address. On the other hand, the least frequently addressed issues were, in order:

1. Relocation trauma
2. Residents' participation in facility governance
3. Medicaid discrimination
4. Boarding home standards
5. Mental health needs of long-term care residents
6. The upgrading of nursing home staff.

With the exception of mental health needs of long-term care residents, these were also among the issues perceived as more difficult to address.

The data thus suggest two possible explanations concerning the ombudsmen's perceived problem focus. It may be interpreted that ombudsmen came to perceive those areas of most frequent contact as less difficult to handle, or, conversely, that they indeed tend to concentrate more activity in areas that are objectively less difficult to address. It should be noted in addition that the issues identified as those most frequently addressed are the very areas in which general ombudsman activity is associated: rights, regulations, and public education. Those issues perceived as less frequently tackled, and more difficult to meet, involve areas exclusively related to long-term care; hence perhaps the greater difficulty of an ombudsman mechanism in its initial development is to cope with and resolve specific long-term care problems.

An analysis of the frequency and perceived difficulty of dealing with complaints at the facility level reveals the opposite trend: with the exception of one item, there seems to be a general positive correlation between the frequency and difficulty of long-term care facility complaints.

The problem or complaint found in the national study to be most often confronted by the ombudsman program is the quality of food and nutrition in the long-term care facility. This complaint is seen by ombudsmen to be one of the least difficult to resolve. The remaining complaint items reveal the opposite trend. The more often a complaint arises, the more difficult it is generally seen to be. The following complaints, dealt with in descending order of frequency, were found to constitute the four most difficult to resolve: poor quality of health care, protection of personal property, administrative expeditiousness, and deficient personal care service. Personal allowances and facility sanitation complaints occur less often and are perceived to be less than moderately difficult. Complaints of residents' interpersonal relations arise with only moderate frequency, and are perceived to be less than moderately difficult. Environmental safety as a problem is perceived to be the least difficult and the least frequent of all the complaint areas listed.

New York City Perspective

The New York City study provided the opportunity for a closer look at the complaint handling and complaint resolution process. During the first half of 1980, contacts with 12,855 patients resulted in 933 documented complaints. An average of 1.9 complaints was recorded per standard three-hour ombudsman visit in a facility. Of all complaints received, 61 percent, or 567, were resolved within the month in which they were lodged. The majority of the complaints were, as in the national survey, in the areas of health care, environment/sanitation, food, and administration. Issues of patients' rights, finances, interpersonal relations, and legality of procedures were less often voiced. In order to determine what problems were seen as the most difficult to deal with by the ombudsmen, both volunteer ombudsmen and facility staff were asked to identify, in descending order, the three most difficult to resolve.

There were two domains where differences between groups

concerning problem severity proved to be significant: food/nutrition and financial. The remaining areas showed no significant differences. It is noted that both ombudsmen and long-term care staff believed issues of food and nutrition to be the number one ranking problem, but the former assigned it a significantly higher level of "resolution difficulty" than the latter.

That is, ombudsmen separated out issues of food/nutrition from other problems, whereas long-term care staff did not make such a sharp distinction. On the other hand, long-term care staff believed financial issues to be significantly more difficult to resolve. Both groups considered issues of health care and interpersonal relations to be among the top five ranking problems that resist resolution. Ombudsmen included, however, patients' rights and administrative issues in this cluster as well, whereas staff did not.

There was close agreement between groups that complaints relating to enviromental conditions and legal aspects of institutional life are not so difficult to solve. It bears consideration that when long-term care staff views of problems were broken down by staff category, directors of social services emerged as having views most consistent with those of the ombudsmen.

What complaints are most likely to recur? Having learned that 91.7 percent of volunteer ombudsmen believed that certain complaints are apt to surface again after having been "resolved," volunteers were asked to choose, in descending order, the three types of complaints most likely to be repeated. The eight problem categories are quite similar to those assigned when resolution difficulty was at issue. Like the local-level information in the national survey, there was a positive association between the recurring nature of certain categories of complaints (food/nutrition, health care, patients' rights, and interpersonal relations) and their resolution difficulty: problems that are less likely to recur (legal, financial, environmental, and administrative) are less likely to be considered troublesome. As expected, patients and problem identification by means of self-observation represented the primary sources for the discovery of long-term care grievances. Two complaint sources assigned secondary importance ("occasional" to "rare") were relatives of patients and nursing home staff. A tertiary cluster of complaint elicitors included residents' councils, nursing home administrators, and family councils, but their contributions to the identification of patient problems had been, indeed, minimal.

Accuracy and Reliability of Residents' Complaints

More than four of every ten volunteer ombudsmen (40.9 percent) estimated that one half to three quarters of complaints received from patients are generally accurate. An additional 22.7 percent offered estimates of 75.0 percent to 90 percent, suggesting that more often than not complaints prove to be legitimate.

Volunteer ombudsmen utilized various approaches to determine the legitimacy of a resident's complaint. The most popular verification procedures have been personal observation and approaching professional staff other than the administrator, such as nurses and social workers. A second set of procedures used "moderately often" included talking with the ombudsman's supervisory staff, questioning other residents or relatives, questioning the administrator, questioning nonprofessional staff (aides and orderlies), and using written ombudsman resources. Ombudsmen "seldom or never" made contact with external regulatory agencies or legal agencies. Finally, ombudsmen placed little value in accepting residents' complaints at face value.

Conclusion

Notwithstanding the unequivocal mandate of the Older Americans Act, which assigns greater weight to the mediative and advocate functions of the ombudsman role, the three major respondent groups at the national level did not arrive at a common interpretation of what the ombudsman is supposed to do. Ombudsmen volunteers do not conform to the legislative role prescription as they tend to slip into a therapeutic range of service behaviors. Highest on the list of priorities of the New York City ombudsmen were qualities such as warmth, caring and concern, and, to a lesser extent, the classical attributes of diplomacy and objectivity. They bear little relationship to the determined and tough-minded advocate. True, though the therapeutic helping role is elevated to primacy, the possibility of engaging in confrontational advocacy strategies is not entirely ruled out. It is demoted instead to a lower level of importance.

Data further revealed that ombudsman program volunteers and long-term care staff do not agree in their views of how to put into operation the ombudsman concept in old age institutions. While facility staff confirm the importance of the therpeutic mode, they fail to differentiate between this approach and that of the impartial mediator. This uncertainty coupled with their rejection of the advocate stance may explain much of their ultimate resistance to the ombudsman concept. Ombudsmen are thus permitted to enter the facilities, but they are not necessarily welcomed. They are treated at times with a mixture of lukewarm sympathy and curiosity. At other times, they are given the cold shoulder of indifference. In sum, they are not viewed by facilities staff as critical or essential actors. Furthermore, the instutitonalized aged do not appear able to comprehend the idea of an impartial mediator or middleman working within the institution. Rather, they perceive external visitors as taking on some kind of partisan stance whether it be therapeutic or adversarial in nature.

Beyond the philosophical polemics about the essence of the ombudsman role there is an emerging plethora of patients' problems, grievances, and complaints. They are the complex, dull, and often intractable realities with which ombudsmen must contend. Whichever way they turn to tackle such reality, it does not appear to be consistent with the classical definitions of this type of redress mechanism. Perhaps an external agent like the ombudsman is needed to contend with the surplus formalization, the institutional impersonality of the nursing home. Yet the advocate concept is viewed as subversive, and the classical, impartial mediator does not seem to display enough of the humanistic qualities so critical to the most vulnerable of the nation's elderly.

It is obvious, then, that the long-term care system has not yet come to terms with the ombudsman role. Given the fact that it lacks sufficient formal empowerment to make its presence properly noticed, does it obtain results? Is the volunteer model effective? This is the subject of chapter 6.

CHAPTER SIX
Do Ombudsman Programs Get Results?

A series of effectiveness and impact measures was developed to determine the extent to which the ombudsman program meets its intended objectives and brings about a measure of improvement in the life of nursing home residents. Four major respondent groups were interviewed:

1. The providers (volunteer ombudsmen and professional staff of the state and local ombudsman programs)
2. The beneficiaries (long-term care facilities residents, in New York City only)
3. Service observers (the aging interest network, long-term care staff, and commissioners of human services)
4. The sponsors (the community board of auspice in New York City).

Providers, sponsors, and observers were questioned as to the degree of success the ombudsmen had realized in meeting ten program issues spelled out in the perceived effectiveness scale and nine impact areas in the perceived impact scale first described in chapter 3. The scales consisted of the following items:

Perceived Effectiveness Scale Items
1. Assist in protecting rights
2. Establish a speedy complaint resolution mechanism
3. Propose changes in policy/regulations
4. Increase communication between staff and residents
5. Establish better community/nursing home relations

6. Improve day-to-day life of residents
7. Provide information for legislators
8. Prevent recurrence of deficiencies
9. Alert staff to patients' needs
10. Support changes in policies/regulations

Perceived Impact Scale Items

1. Severity of problems
2. General quality of services
3. Accountability of staff actions
4. Degree of patient participation in life decisions
5. Quality of nursing home/community relations
6. Quality of relations among staff
7. Satisfaction of residents with services
8. Overall social climate
9. Quality of staff/resident relations

Measures of provider and observer responses along two hypothesized dimensions of program effectiveness and two dimensions of program impact were derived by means of the judgments of an expert panel. Panel members were asked to judge the "degree of fit" of the original series of ten effectiveness issues and nine impact areas within three proposed effectiveness dimensions (1: policy/planning; 2: organizational/programmatic; and 3: relationship/social interactive) and two proposed impact dimensions (a: technical service; and b: social). The Student-Neuman-Keuls procedure allowed the identification of homogeneous subsets for items at the $p < .05$ level, and ultimately the assignment of three effectiveness items and four impact items to four goal-attainment dimensions.

Cronbach standardized item alphas of .92 and .81 were obtained in the national study and .81 and .88 in the New York City survey for the perceived impact and effectiveness scales. Reliability coefficients of .41 and .45 obtained for the multiple item dimensional measures were deemed acceptable in light of the limited number of items in each of these subscales. Internal correlation coefficients between all perceived effectiveness items ranged from .44 to .77 in the national and .15 to .74 in the New York City studies. The correlation matrix for the perceived impact scale included coefficients ranging from .41 to .66 and from −.07 to .64 in the abovementioned studies.

A composite measure of "experienced" effectiveness was also developed and administered to elderly users of the ombudsman services designated as program beneficiaries. This five-item scale allowed aged residents the opportunity to assess whether the ombudsman they spoke to was sensitive, respectful, interested in their problem, competent to deal with their problem, and accountable, that is, able to keep them informed of results. High reliability was also achieved for this scale (alpha coefficient = .91). Internal correlation coefficients between items ranged from .57 to .89.

Strengths and Weaknesses—

The State Ombudsman's View

State ombudsmen are the only public officials armed with a holistic perspective on the ombudsman program's operation at different levels of government. They were asked, therefore, to make a comparative assessment of the program's relative effectiveness and impact at the state and local levels. More specifically, they weighted the extent of program success in addressing the following issues extrapolated from the perceived effectiveness scale:

1. Proposing changes in nursing home policies and regulations
2. Establishing better relationships between community and nursing home groups
3. Providing information for legislators and program planners for bringing about changes in long-term care
4. Establishing a speedy mechanism for resolving resident complaints
5. Assisting in the protection of patients' rights
6. Alerting nursing home staff and administration to patient needs.

This group of respondents claimed that the state-level ombudsman program achieved greatest effectiveness in providing information for legislators and long-term care program planners, closely followed by their capacity to assist in the protection of residents' rights. Moderate success rates were reported for the establishment of a complaint resolution mechanism, the alerting of nursing home staff to patients' needs, and the establishment of better relationships between the nursing home and the community. Less than moderate effectiveness was indicated for the state-level ombudsman program in proposing changes in nursing home policies and regulations.

The same issues considered for effectiveness at the local ombudsman program level revealed differences and similarities with the preceding state-level observations. Greatest effectiveness was realized in the alerting of nursing home staff to patient needs. Assisting in the protection of residents' rights, on the other hand, retained its second-place position as noted for state-level ombudsman programs. Efforts at establishing better community/nursing home relations and complaint resolution mechanisms were seen to have been moderately successful. The provision of information and the making of policy change proposals, on the other hand, were viewed as activities less effectively carried out at the local level.

Tests of significance revealed significant differences in the perceived effectiveness rates when viewing selected issue areas at both state and local level. The nursing home ombudsman program was found to be significantly more effective at the state level in proposing changes in nursing home policies and regulations, and in providing information for legislators and long-term care program planners. Conversely, the local-level ombudsman program was viewed as significantly more effective than its state-level counterpart in alerting nursing home staff and administration to patients' needs. The remaining issue areas were perceived by the respondents to be equally well handled at both state and local levels of the nursing home program.

State ombudsmen were subsequently asked about the programs' relative impact in four items extrapolated from the perceived impact scale:

1. The accountability of staff actions in nursing homes
2. The quality of nursing home/community relations
3. The quality of relations among staff in nursing homes
4. The quality of staff/resident relations in nursing homes.

State ombudsmen assigned identical values for the ordering of impact items at both the state and local levels. Increasing the accountability of staff in nursing homes was seen to be the area most positively affected at both program levels, followed by upgrading the quality of nursing home/community relations, staff/residents relations, and relations among staff in nursing homes.

Comparative T-tests revealed, however, that there were significant differences in the relative magnitude of impact at the respective program levels. Specifically, the local nursing home ombudsman program was seen to achieve significantly greater influence in improving the quality of nursing home/community relations and staff/residents relations than the state-level program. The accountability of staff actions in nursing homes, on the other hand, was seen to be positively affected at equivalent levels at both state and local levels, whereas the quality of relations among staff in nursing homes was least likely to be altered in a positive manner at either the state or local level of the nursing home ombudsman program.

These findings suggest, therefore, that areas related to the establishment and enforcement of patients' rights, including legislative influence, are most effectively considered and influenced at the state level. The more immediate, interpersonal issues emerging out of the day-to-day operations of the long-term care facility, on the other hand, are seen to be most successfully dealt with by the mediational interventions of a local ombudsman program.

Effectiveness and Impact

The National Survey

Do local volunteer ombudsmen get results when they respond to residents' complaints? Do they properly identify latent and emerging problems? Does their presence in long-term care facilities contribute to enhancing the quality of patient care?

Four scales already mentioned—the issue effectiveness scale, the complaint effectiveness scale, the perceived effectiveness scale, and the perceived impact scale—were utilized in the national study to respond to these evaluative questions. The major overall finding was that the three survey groups—the aging interest group, the human services commissioners, and the long-term providers—hardly agreed on any of their answers. The issue effectiveness scale inquired how well ombudsmen deal with residents' rights, issues of abuse and neglect of patients, enforcement of nursing home regulations, arbitrary or discriminatory practices in Medicaid reimbursement, quality of the nursing home staff, residents relocation trauma, development and enforcement of boarding homes standards, consumer education relating to long-term care, development of alternatives to institutionalization, abuse or misappropriation of residents' funds, and facilitation of residents' participation in the governance of the nursing home facility. A reliability coefficient of .92 was obtained for the scale with interitem coefficients ranging from .31 to .77.

Data revealed that the aging interest group perceived moderate effectiveness in the areas of residents' rights, abuse of residents, and enforcement of regulations with all the remaining issues achieving only slight effectiveness. The human services commissioners considered the ombudsman program moderately effective only on residents' rights, with other measures recording slightly to hardly effective ratings. The long-term care providers emerged as having the most negative view of program effectiveness, assigning minimal levels of effectiveness to all program efforts. Intergroup differences were all significant at the p < .01 level.

The trend discovered earlier in which the aging interest group was the most supportive of the ombudsman program, the human services commissioners moderately supportive, and the long-term care providers least supportive in their estimation of program value, was repeated in these findings.

When considering relative item effectiveness in the ratings of issue efficacy, all three groups viewed the ombudsman program as most effective in meeting issues of residents' rights and abuse of residents. Conversely, the majority of the respondent groups considered the ombudsman program to be least effective in regard to boarding home standards and the upgrading of nursing home staff. Interestingly, these last two issues were rated by the state ombudsmen themselves as the two most difficult items to address.

The complaint effectiveness scale measured a range of facility-level issues or complaints. The scale consisted of the following items:

1. Food/nutrition
2. Administration
3. Environmental safety
4. Facility sanitation
5. Interpersonal relations (residents)
6. Personal care (help with washing, dressing)
7. Health care
8. Personal allowance
9. Protection of personal property.

A standardized item alpha of .94 was obtained confirming higher reliability. Between items, correlation coefficients ranged from .49 to .81. As in the previous survey measure, each internal scale item obtained significant group mean differences in analysis of variance. A consistent pattern of responses by the three major groups was obtained in this scale as well: the aging interest group rated the programs' effectiveness in dealing with the complaint item the highest; human services respondents assigned middle-range scores; and the long term care providers, the lowest scores. Intergroup scores indicated, on the other hand, that all respondents considered the handling of such complaints by the ombudsman program to be at best only moderately effective, and more often than not, only slightly effective.

Within-group differences were discerned for the three major responding groups as well. Both human services commissioners and long-term care providers considered complaints about food to be the ones most effectively treated at the facility level. On the other hand, the aging interest group viewed problems in health care as those most effectively met by the ombudsman program. Health care was seen by the human services commissioners and long-term care providers to be less successfully met.

The clearest finding from this scale, however, is the magnitude of each group's effectiveness ratings. The lowest rated complaint area among the aging interest group was higher than the most highly rated such area among the human services providers. Similarly, in descending order and except for one item, the lowest rated of the complaint areas among the human services commissioners was more highly rated than the complaint considered by the long-term care providers to be the most effectively addressed by the ombudsman program. These findings thus reinforce the trend that has been unfolding throughout this analysis: one in which the aging interest group is most supportive of the ombudsman program, the long term care providers least supportive, and the human services commissioners taking a position midpoint between the two other groups.

The perceived effectiveness scale provided additional reinforcement for the response trend. Respondents were asked to rate on an interval scale how successful the ombudsman program has been in carrying out a range of programmatic tasks. The scale included the following nine items:

1. Propose changes in nursing home policies and regulations
2. Establish better relationships between community and nursing home groups
3. Provide information for legislators and program planners for bringing about changes in long-term care
4. Establish a speedy mechanism for resolving residents' complaints
5. Assist in the protection of residents' rights
6. Alert nursing home staff and administration to patients' needs
7. Develop a statewide ombundsman network
8. Develop an information clearinghouse
9. Public education on long-term care

The items include reference to facility-level, state-program level, and policy-level issues. Analysis of variance revealed significant group mean differences for each of the nine scale items as well as the summary index measure.

As in the previous scales, the aging interest group indicated that the ombudsman program had been most successful, and the human services commissioners accorded more success than did the long-term care providers. Unlike the previous scales, there was virtually no variation in the relative rankings of items within each group. All groups found the program most successful in protecting patients' rights and in establishing a complaint mechanism. Low levels of success were perceived by the three major respondent groups in the following areas: development of an information clearinghouse, public education on long-term care, and proposing policy changes in long-term care.

The results thus indicate that despite differences in magnitude in the absolute effectiveness scores, respondents saw the greatest ombudsman program success in the performance of intended ombudsman functions, and the least success in ancillary public relations functions or partisan policy advocacy. These findings further suggest that while there may be significant differences across groups as to the degree of success realized by this program in its efforts to assure quality long-term care, the ombudsman has most clearly affirmed an image closer to its classical roots.

Respondents were finally asked to indicate the degree of impact attained by the ombudsman program in four areas of the long-term care delivery system (the items of the perceived impact scale were presented earlier in this chapter in the section on research procedures). The findings indicate that all the respondents perceived at the least the virtual absence of any program influence, and at most, slightly positive levels of influence.

Significant differences were obtained in analysis of variance for intergroup mean scores on all four individual scale items. Again, the lowest impact score indicated by the aging interest group was greater than the highest score granted by the long-term care providers. The human service commissioners fell between the two other groups in regard to their ratings of ombudsman program impact.

Within-group rankings also revealed differences between the perceptions of long-term care providers and of the other groups regarding the influence of the program. Long-term care providers perceived the highest levels to be in improving the quality of staff/resident relations in the nursing home, an area viewed by the other two respondent groups as having been only marginally affected. Conversely, the long-term care providers assigned a lower rating to the level of accountability of staff actions in nursing homes, the very area considered by both the aging interest group and the human services commissioners to have been most improved by the actions of the ombudsman program.

The response trend in which long-term care providers were distinguishable from the other respondent groups both in their discordant views of ombudsman program components and in their lower estimation of the overall value of the ombudsman program was reaffirmed.

Correlated *T*-tests were also performed for each possible pairing of the three major respondent groups, on each summary scale score. The findings underscored the trends that have been identified thus far. For each scale, the aging interest group indicated the most highly effective rating, the human services commissioners, the next highest, and the long-term care providers, the least effective rating. Similarly, the aging interest group indicated that the ombudsman program was most influential, the human services commissioners, the second most positive impact, and the long-term care providers, the least positive influence. In essence, only the aging interest group stands out in its positive evaluations. All others have a considerable distance to go toward recognizing any noticeable merit in the nursing home ombudsman program.

The New York City Survey

The New York City study initially targeted its program performance measures on five respondent groups: the three long-term care staff professional groups—nursing home administrators, directors of nursing, and directors of social services—plus the volunteer ombudsmen and a sample of residents, namely, the actual service beneficiaries. Supplementing the effectiveness and impact scales used in the national survey were four single-item performance measures, each rated on a five-point scale:

"Does the program fill a service gap in long-term care facilities?"
"What priority do you assign to the continuation of the program?"
"How would you rate the overall effectiveness of the program?"
"Has the presence of the ombudsman made a difference in the lives of the residents?"

Correlations obtained among all goal attainment measures were significant, ranging from .24 between "difference in patient life" and "extent of gap filling," to .77, between "perceived effectiveness" and "change in patients' lives." Positive relationships at the $p < .05$ level or greater existed between all measures.

Summary statistics and analysis of variance across the five respondent groups revealed considerable agreement on the extent of achieved program efficacy. Significant variance between groups appeared for one single-item goal attainment measure only: "the difference the program has made in the patients' lives."

The high level of intergroup consistency was further emphasized when reviewing the mean scores of volunteer ombudsmen and facility staff across the entire range of perceived effectiveness and perceived impact scale items. Significant group variance at the $p < .05$ level was found for only one of the ten program effectiveness issues ("improving the day-to-day life of residents"). In this case, volunteer ombudsmen believed that they had achieved significantly greater success than long-term care staff generally, and nursing home administrators in particular, were willing to concede. Group views varied significantly, again at the $p < .05$ level, for only two of the nine areas of possible impact: (1) "The severity of problems in nursing homes" and (2) "The quality of staff/resident relations." In the case of the first issue it was apparently the negative views of the directors of nursing that pulled the groups apart, whereas for the second issue it was the critical judgment of the directors of social services.

Long-term care staff agreed that the program achieved "moderate" to "low" degrees of success with a tendency for directors of social services to be more negative about ombudsman performance than other facility staff. The former were not fully convinced that the program is filling a "service gap" in long-term care but acknowledged that this may be partially the case. In looking to the future, they believed program continuation to be of "moderate" priority. Staff was noncommittal when asked to assess overall program effectiveness. Similarly, staff means for perceived effectiveness and impact measures indicated that program effort was only "slightly successful" and had been from "no impact" to "slightly positive" impact respectively.

Residents who acknowledged having used the ombudsman

service aligned themselves with long-term care staff in their estimates of the extent to which the program has made a difference in the lives of the institutionalized aged. Both respondent groups accorded the program "moderate" success in this respect. Volunteer ombudsmen, on the other hand, believed the program to have made a measurably greater difference in patients' lives. These volunteers were, however, in close accord with facility staff concerning perceptions of program effectiveness and impact.

Data indicate that 43.8 percent of service users were "very satisfied" with the way in which the ombudsman handled their complaints while an additional 26.1 percent were "fairly satisfied." Only 17.1 percent of actual users registered feelings of dissatisfaction on this issue (13.0 percent were not sure as to their feelings). Among those who were dissatisfied, insufficient responses by the volunteers to their requests for aid were most often given as explanation. Furthermore, among patients who had presented grievances to a volunteer ombudsman, 43.5 percent believed that the problems were solved, 39.1 percent thought they were not, and 17.4 percent were not sure. When patients were asked to assess their personal experiences with the ombudsman, using the five-item experienced effectiveness scale, agreement again emerged that a relatively high level of effectiveness was achieved. Analysis of individual scale items indicated, however, that ombudsman volunteers were considerably more likely to be seen as "sensitive," "respectful," and "interested" than "competent" or "accountable." When actual users of the service were asked to describe the ways in which the volunteer ombudsman had made life better for older people in the home, there was almost unanimous agreement that the effect was an individual one, on a case-by-case basis rather than collective in nature. Finally, among patients who expressed an evaluative opinion, there was strong endorsement for the idea that the ombudsman should continue visiting their facility in the future.

The perceptions of volunteer ombudsmen were very similar to those of long-term care staff along the program effectiveness and impact dimensions mentioned in the section on research procedures and described in Appendix B. The method by which these dimensions were validated has been discussed. The "policy/planning" dimension implies that ombudsman-initiated change is more likely to have collective or systemic rather than individual consequences for long-term institutional care. The "relationship/social interactive" dimension reflects interpersonal or socializing consequences of ombudsman activity. The "technical service" dimension reflects general programmatic and organizational efforts of ombudsmen, whereas the "social" dimension focuses on ombudsman impact on general qualitative interactions between individuals. A significant difference between providers and observers was found for only one dimension—the "relationship/social interactive" one. Interestingly, long-term care staff believed that the ombudsman program has been more effective in establishing better community/nursing home relations than the volunteers themselves.

It is worthy of note that three of the original ten effectiveness items judged by the expert panel not to merit inclusion in a hypothesized "organizational/programmatic dimension" were accorded considerably higher levels of attainment than the actual validated dimensions. This was the case for both external agents and long-term care staff. The high scores for these program effectiveness items—(1) alerting staff to patient needs; (2) assisting in the protection of residents' rights; and (3) establishing a speedy complaint resolution mechanism—seemed to indicate that the ombudsman program was considerably more successful in establishing specific piecemeal procedures and processes in the facilities than in bringing about structural changes in the long-term care system or improving social relationships between individuals and groups in the same context.

Members of the community advisory boards in New York City were also invited to express their views about the programs' results. Their overall sense was that ombudsmen had achieved "moderate success" across a range of issues, but their highest praise was reserved to three of them: introducing limited changes in individual facilities, establishing a working mechanism for complaint resolution, and improving the general quality of life of the residents. They perceived the ombudsmen volunteers to be lacking in knowing how to bring about fundamental systemic changes in the makeup of institutional care and in proposing new policies and regulations.

Analysis of secondary data of sponsor agencies provided an additional qualitative perspective of program performance. Repeatedly stressed during field interviews with community network representatives in New York City was the success of ombudsman program personnel in: (1) opening nursing homes to the community and thus elevating community consciousness around the long-term care issue; (2) instituting a degree of "personal advocacy" in which one-to-one relationships between ombudsman and residents' are developed and maintained; (3) identifying problems which when serious enough are passed on to the proper regulatory authority; (4) enlisting a group of citizen volunteers who are sensitive, concerned, and persistent in their efforts; and (5) establishing throughout the community a degree of integrity, respect, and political savvy that is unusual for a program still young in terms of actual operation. The fact that the program existed at all and had a presence in a number of facilities was felt by many to represent an accomplishment of no small order.

It is important to recognize that while the community sponsors and salaried program staff supervisors acknowledged that there had been more limited program influence at the system's level than at the level of the individual resident, reference was made to two specific victories in which collective improvements had been realized.

In the first instance, a high number of complaints in health care, patients' rights, and environment/sanitation had continually resisted resolution in one facility despite the efforts of the two assigned ombudsmen. Subsequent to consultations with, and promises of support from, the New York State Nursing Home Patient Ombudsman, the executive director of the ombudsman program sponsoring agency (Community Council of Greater New York) and the chairperson of the community's Committee of Auspice, a comprehensive report was presented to the New York State Office of Health Systems Management's patients' advocate and its director of long-term care services, the agency having statutory responsibility for ensuring quality care for institutionalized patients and residents. Despite the reaction of the facility's administration, the Office of Health Systems Management (OHSM) supported the findings of the ombudsman program and took appropriate action. The result was a measurable improvement not for one patient, but for residents throughout the facility in terms of better food, a cleaner environment, and better overall care.

The second victory involved a situation described in the February 1980 issue of the *Ombudsnews,* the official newsletter of the New York City nursing home patient ombudsman program (the names of the facility in question and of those individuals involved have been changed to maintain anonymity):

> Last month, HEW notified Oak Tree Home that its Medicare license, due to expire on January 31 would not be renewed. The cancellation of Medicare automatically cuts off Medicaid payments to the facility, and, in effect, forces the closing of the facility, and the relocation of all the residents to new facilities. John Doe, Oak Tree's Ombudsman, noticed that many of Oak Tree's residents were upset and disconcerted over HEW's decision.
>
> The Ombudsman Program Director brought this situation to the attention of the local Committee of Auspice in January. The Committee agreed that the residents should have a right to participate in any decision affecting their continued residency or transfer from Oak Tree. NHPOP's position is that the residents of any facility have "property interests" in their facility, interests which include the right to a fair hearing before any transfer. While HEW had informed the facility's administration of the cancellation of its Medicare license and its fair hearing rights, the residents were not given the same right. NHPOP did not dispute the longstanding deficiencies recorded by OHSM's surveyers, but argued that apart from the certain trauma of transfer to many residents which could jeopardize their lives, the residents would get little choice in the facilities to which they would be transferred, and that they would be deprived of the friendships and special cultural benefits that Oak Tree provided.

The Committee felt that closing Oak Tree would be inappropriate without exhausting other remedies more benevolent to the residents. Tom Smith of the Legal Aid Society agreed to represent those residents wishing to participate in the facility's fair hearing proceedings.

John Doe and Jim Wilson, the local Field Supervisor, visited Oak Tree several times and discussed HEW's decision with many of the residents. The residents were eager to stop the transfers and asked NHPOP to contact Legal Aid on their behalf and arrange to have Legal Aid assist them. To strengthen the residents' case, the NHPOP became co-plaintiff with the residents in this proceeding.

Legal Aid successfully obtained a temporary restraining order in U.S. District Court, delaying the termination of Oak Tree's Medicare license. The order guaranteed adequate time for Oak Tree to reach agreement on a voluntary receivership, thus insuring the residents their continued stay at Oak Tree. During a second hearing on the case ten days later, the court was impressed with the improved conditions of Oak Tree under the new receiver. HEW and OHSM conceded that conditions were considerably improved, and the Court then extended the restraining order for an additional thirty days, provided the facility and receiver enter into a formal contract.[1]

The court action and a subsequent court appearance led to a settlement encompassing several important concessions on the part of the new voluntary receiver. The "Oak Tree" case was in fact one of the largest resident-initiated cases in New York State's history. It established the right of institutionalized individuals to participate in the decisions that determine the policies governing a facility's operations and in determining who will actually administer those policies.

Changes as described above have been the exception rather than the rule for the ombudsman program. They did establish, however, an important precedent for the long-term care field.

Program Awareness Among Nursing Home Residents

The effectiveness of the ombudsman program is, to a large extent, contingent on the realization of its existence among nursing home residents. In order to assess the level of achieved program awareness, residents in fifteen New York City participating facilities were asked as to their knowledge of the presence of the volunteer ombudsman. Three awareness probes were made: (1) "Have you heard of the volunteer ombudsman who talks to people living in this home?"; (2) "Do you know about the volunteer with the green badge who visits here?"; and (3) "Have you heard of [name of ombudsman] who comes to talk to people on this floor?" Less than one third, or 27.6 percent, of the total sample responded affirmatively to at least one of the three probes, suggesting a relatively low level of information about the program. Upon further questioning (of the "program-aware" group, 16.0 percent claimed to know the location of the ombudsman's office, 22.4 percent stated they knew when the ombudsman was supposed to be in the facility, and 8.2 percent maintained they knew where to call the ombudsman when he/she was not there. Thus a relatively low level of "specific" awareness appeared among the most aware group.

It is significant to add that males were considerably more likely to have heard of the ombudsman than females, and residents of proprietary homes significantly more so than those in voluntary facilities. Furthermore, the least educated (less than a high school education) were significantly less likely to have heard of the ombudsman and similarly less likely to feel they should tell someone about their problems when they come up.

Resident awareness of the patients' bill of rights (State Hospital Code Sections 730.17 and 740.14) which by law is a document requiring posting in all health care facilities, was highly correlated with an awareness of the ombudsman's presence. This finding becomes especially noteworthy when coupled with data pointing out that only one in three among the total sample acknowledged ever having heard of this document. In addition, it was the patients 75 years of age and older and the less educated patients who were less likely to know of this document's existence, though in the case of the latter this tendency did not reach a significant level.

While 27.6 percent of all residents interviewed reported knowing of the volunteer ombudsman in their facility, only 9 percent indicated having actually reported complaints to the ombudsman. Problems presented were most often related to health care, food/nutrition, and patients' rights issues, in that order. Furthermore, data indicated that in most instances, complaints were activated at the initiative of the volunteer ombudsman, or some other professional agent rather than that of the residents.

Data indicated that 68 percent of the volunteer ombudsmen found that residents "often" express fear of reprisal by long-term care staff when lodging complaints. An additional 28 percent maintained that this is "sometimes" the case. About 20 percent of the residents who knew of the program admitted that they have worried about facility staff being angry with them if they were to tell the ombudsman about a problem. It is worth noting that this fear of staff criticism or retaliation was acknowledged significantly more often among proprietary home than voluntary home patients. Similarly, 19 percent of the total patient sample admitted to having held back from talking to nursing home employees about a problem since they have been living there. Again, it is the proprietary home patient who appeared significantly more likely to have held back than the voluntary facility patient. These data become particularly meaningful when coupled with the finding that proprietary patients rated the quality of care in their facilities to be significantly worse than that of their peers living in the not-for-profit facilities.

Less than half of the residents interviewed (43.8 percent) acknowledged that they had always told someone about a complaint or problem when it was bothering them. They revealed that they did not always verbalize these concerns because they felt it would be useless or futile (54.9 percent), because they feared retaliation (19.6 percent), or because they did not trust the staff enough (13.7 percent).

Nursing home patients underscored that the ombudsman was rarely the first person to whom they would direct complaints. Thirty-seven percent of the resident sample considered a nurse the best person to complain to, 25.6 percent mentioned the social worker, and 16.3 percent suggested it should be the administrator. Only 6.9 percent turned first to relatives, and barely one percent turned to others from the outside such as ombudsmen. While residents in long-term care facilities had doubts about telling institutional employees their problems, the latter, nevertheless, remained the primary source for personal aid.

Role Orientation and Program Efficacy

Chapter 5 reviewed the range of ombudsman interventive behaviors and examined the frequency and circumstances that prompt volunteers to identify with either the mediating, the advocacy, or the therapeutic role orientations. The New York study went a step further by inquiring whether there is a relationship between any of the three role patterns and a discernible measure of program success. It found that long-term care staff associated the attainment of higher levels of all categories of program effectiveness and impact with the ombudsman who functions in the classical vein as an impartial intermediary. The therapeutic supporter—one who emphasizes the expression of friendly concern and caring—was correlated with both greater technical and social impact in long-term care. No such correlative trend was found between the advocate role and program performance.

In the case of the volunteer ombudsman, the relationship between role perceptions and views of goal attainment was less differentiated. As ombudsmen perceived themselves to be more like advocates (that is, as adversaries and politically partisan), they were more likely to believe that the program had achieved higher levels of policy/planning effectiveness. The relationship between the advocate role and the rating of social interactive effectiveness was similarly positive but fell short of significance. Ombudsmen significantly associated the therapeutic role with social interactive effectiveness. The therapeutic function was also positively correlated with policy/planning effectiveness through the relationship did not achieve statistical significance. Ombudsmen's perception of the mediative function approached significant associations with both social interactive effectiveness and social impact.

In sum, then, ombudsmen did not exclude a specific role from the possibility of getting results. They were implicitly stating that all role approaches are equally valid and useful. Their eclecticism thus reflected a broader role conception than the one espoused by the long-term care staff. After considering the goal-attainment merits of the three ombudsman role orientations, an analysis of the volunteer and the professional ombudsman personnel patterns constituted the next logical step in the inquiry.

Voluntarism or Professionalism

In order to maximize coverage of nursing home facilities across their entire geographical domain, and to facilitate greater local program development, many state ombudsman programs enlist the aid of volunteers. New York and Connecticut have made extensive use of volunteer "advocates" at the local level, and Georgia was planning to do so at the time of this study. An alternate approach, on the other hand, is one that focuses primarily upon paid professional staff as in the case of New Jersey. The survey thus went to inqure about the status of ombudsman program personnel patterns.

State ombudsmen reported that while slightly less than half of the states utilized mainly a salaried professional base, the majority of the programs reflected varying mixes of professionals and volunteers. Only one in ten state ombudsman programs reported a dominant volunteer staff.

The implications of such different staffing patterns include on the one hand the potentially lower status accorded the volunteer-based programs by the long-term care providers, and hence lower acceptance of its goals and function. Conversely, the responsibility of salaried professional nursing home ombudsmen to their employer could threaten their own impartiality and objectivity, factors characteristic of the classical ombudsman model. There are trade-offs inherent therefore in each personnel pattern as program effectiveness is concerned.

The preferred future personnel makeup as reported by state ombudsmen indicates a regression to the mean. The frequency distribution showed less polarization and more general acceptance of the need for a mix of paid staff and volunteers. There was no clear consensus toward a preferred volunteer or preferred salaried staff pattern, thus leading to a range of interpretations rather than to a single, consistent trend.

Some of the ambivalence regarding the use of volunteers transcends strategic and philosophical trade-offs and stems from the simple difficulty in recruiting nonsalaried individuals. State ombudsmen were queried, therefore, as to the importance of a range of factors in the recruitment and retention of volunteers in the ombudsman program. Respondents were asked to rank the following items: the availability of stipends, the volunteers' desire to help, supervisory assistance, the quality of training, mutual support available from other volunteers, the amount of power or clout available to the volunteer, and previous advocacy experience, as to their relative importance for the recruitment and for the retention of volunteers. A look at both rankings within each dimension and T-tests comparing each item across the dimensions of recruitment and retention are instructive.

The altruism of volunteers was found to be the foremost factor for their successful recruitment, followed by the quality of training and supervisory assistance. Advocacy experience and mutual support from other volunteers were found to be only moderately important. Least important were stipends and clout available to the volunteer. The factors that foster the retention of volunteers over time were found to be similarly distributed with minimal variations. Supervisory assistance was identified as the single most important factor in the retention of volunteers, with quality of training slightly edging out volunteers' altruism for the second position. Mutual support and clout were seen to be more important for retention than initial recruitment, and previous advocacy experience as less crucial. The availability of stipends maintained a low rank of importance across both dimensions.

Statistical tests underlined the extent of differential importance assigned to certain items across the dimensions of recruitment and retention. The volunteers' desire to help and previous advocacy experience were significantly more important as recruitment aids than as retention factors. Conversely, supervisory assistance, mutual support, and the amount of clout or power to effect change available to the volunteer were significantly more important as retention aids, as opposed to recruitment factors. Interestingly, the quality of training was seen to be equally important, and the availability of stipends equally unimportant for both the recruitment and the retention of volunteers in the ombudsman program.

The findings suggest, therefore, that volunteer ombudsmen personnel are self-motivated and somewhat activist in orientation. Once recruited, however, altruistic impulse and partisan concern alone do not suffice. Skills acquisition and technical/supervisory support move to the fore as important factors prolonging volunteer service. Even so, the citizen volunteer is not primarily motivated by financial considerations, nor are volunteers deterred by the limitations of power available to them. Members of the New York City community advisory boards of the ombudsman program also identified the volunteers' enthusiasm and altruistic commitment as the program's primary strength. Objectivity and independence of judgment were the next valued attributes. The two most serious shortcomings mentioned were the inadequacy in the level of technical skills or expertise that volunteers bring to the position, and the limited time they can invest in discharging their duties.

Two notes from the field provide a contradictory impression, however, as to the role of training and stipends. The Georgia long-term care ombudsman program is unique in that the state legislation which established the program requires a rigorous training period for both salaried and volunteer staff, namely, the community ombudsmen. In addition, the law mandates that ombudsman personnel pass a comprehensive examination at the conclusion of the training. These provisions were established to upgrade the image and status of the volunteers and to ensure that only qualified individuals represent the program.

One consequence of these rather demanding training requirements was difficulty in the successful recruitment of volunteers as opposed to salaried staff. More lenient training periods were being proposed at the time of the study in selected regions of Georgia in which more flexible guidelines would allow completion of the training over a more extended period of time than was statutorily prescribed. The implication, therefore, is that while quality training is seen as both a recruitment and a retention aid, training that is too rigidly structured and comprehensive may inadvertently deter individuals from assuming the volunteer ombudsman role.

The New York State nursing home ombudsman program reported a variation in the findings concerning stipends. The area ombudsman program whose volunteers have attained the most cohesiveness and who have succeeded in enacting particularly effective advocacy efforts was the one which provides the volunteers with a stipend of $5.00 per hour for four weekly visitation hours. This would suggest that the provision of stipends played a greater role than the survey data suggest. An appropriate explanation would perhaps be that it is not the stipend *per se,* but its symbolic content as official recognition that facilitates more enthusiastic volunteer involvement.

Additional notes from the field highlight some of the risks inherent in a volunteer model: its tendency to oscillate between a confrontational stance and the more innocuous extreme of friendly visiting; a resistance to comply with basic administrative reporting; the formidable opposition orchestrated by the nursing home establishment; and the unrealistic expectations placed upon the volunteers' capacity to effect changes. The debate that evolves from many of these inter-

views seems to center on a minimalist concept of the ombudsman role, one that would restrict the volunteer to watchdogging and alerting a second line of back-up specialists. Other
repondents disagreed: they regard the ombudsman as capable
of encompassing a broader range of interventions than they
have actually been given credit for. Policy analysis and program development are just two of them. The following notes
from field interviews are illustrative of the voluntar-
ism/professionalism debate.

A regional ombudsman in the state of Connecticut saw problems in controlling the action of certain patient advocates. Some,
he believed, do not know the boundary of their responsibilities
and immediately take on a confrontational stance in dealing with
nursing home administrators. They overlook the importance of
establishing a working relationship which is nonadversarial. "Only
the latter can promote lasting and effective results when complaints actually arrive." He conceded, however, that regional
ombudsmen are greatly assisted by the volunteers who serve in
their jurisdictions. If not for them, the regional ombudsman
could not attend to all the problems that surface.

One volunteer patient advocate in the same state confirmed
their independence of action. Mr. L. admitted that he goes over-
board sometimes and exceeds his authority by assuming tasks
well beyond the formal description of his duties. He felt he must
have free reign in what he does or he would find continuing
serving in the program pointless. For instance, he makes bank
deposits for patients, he advises them on financial matters, en-
sures the delivery of publications to patients, and so on. Mr. L.
boasted that he does not record in writing the daily service process. He refuses to do the paper work, and the staff is already
resigned to it: program staff are "able to know well enough about
what I do through my verbal communications." On the other
hand, he is willing to handle complaints on the spot and often
takes calls at home.

Mr. L. praised the ombudsman program as one of the few
where problems once reported get instantaneous attention. Prior
to its inception, simple concerns such as patients with urine-
stained clothing or those who needed eye and teeth examina-

tions were not attended to. "Now a patients' advocate can get such problems resolved quickly." However, a major weakness of the program is its inability to locate enough volunteers. There is not enough incentive. In Mr. L.'s opinion, a nominal compensation in the range of $1,000 a year would ensure more frequent visitations and a more serious attendance at training sessions.

In Mr. L.'s view, the terms "ombudsman" and "advocate" are almost meaningless and are often misunderstood by the people who receive services. He believes he does more than engage in advocacy. "I go beyond the term. My work is all-encompassing: I may both fight to improve a service and provide a shoulder to cry on for a needy patient."

The pool from which volunteers are selected and their motivation to enroll in the program were questioned by the legal services developer for a Northeastern state. He felt that too often the wrong people join the program: some are "busybodies" who want to know the personal problems of others to satisfy their own curiosity. Others come with a tough-minded predisposition, wanting to remove clients from their facilities, and create perpetual warfare with the staff manning those institutions.

The same informant suggested restricting the volunteer to one who simply acts as the eyes and the ears of the program as a whole:

> They should not overstep those boundaries. Too often, however, they are dissatisfied with the limits placed on them and it is virtually impossible to restrain them. They want to act as enforcers. . . . The fact that the state legislature is volunteer-crazy adds to the stress of working with volunteers. Once the honeymoon of enlisting them is over, one soon discovers that there is no such a thing as a free lunch, when it comes to volunteer time contributions. One must take the good with the bad and invest considerably in their training and supervision without any certainty of how much they will give back in services and for how long, given their high burn-out rate.

A state ombudsman for a Northeastern state expressed a similar concern about the ideological framework brought by volunteers. "It is detrimental to the ultimate program objectives," he stated, "when they arrive with the conviction that all nursing homes are bad. They start from a hard-nosed and antagonistic perspective and damage many of the gains already made in initiating rapport with numerous facilities." Their role, he felt, should be instead that of an external, independent listener, and they should not be perceived as ogres entering the facility to destroy it, but as problem-solvers who will sit down and assist both staff and patients. "They have a helping mission to perform, one of nailing down the critical issues. In any event, they are not meant to be an enemy of anyone."

Mr. T., the state ombudsman of a Western state, saw, in turn, both advantages and shortcomings in the use of volunteers. One drawback is that there is a limit to the time they are able to donate, and their turnover rate is high. Salaried professionals, he remarked, do not stay long on their jobs either. Whether volunteers or salaried professionals, ombudsmen seem to perform better in rural than in urban areas because in the latter one finds facilities that are larger, more complex, and more sophisticated. Distances to travel between facilities in rural districts, however, are great, and there are no provisions for reimbursement of transportation. Some individuals run into monthly gas bills of nearly $200, the car's depreciation not considered. Moreover, many of the actions they have to take require long-distance calls to relatives, licensing governmental offices, specialists, and so on. Just getting in touch with the health department, a daily routine in the ombudsman's work, may well require a long-distance call in a rural area. Communication and transportation costs reach prohibitive levels in no time. "It is astonishing that these people accept taking on such an expense. No wonder that the majority end up dropping out in less than a year. How long can they go on subsidizing the program from their own pockets?"

Mr. T. is convinced that the work of the ombudsman is the most difficult in the field of aging. The program hardly backs up its participants with technical resources and updated information, it is underfunded, and it provides no incentives other than the challenge of the job itself. It requires, furthermore, that individuals with often limited training and armed primarily with good will and intuition enter into hostile environments where they are confronted by a powerful and multimillion-dollar industry capable of counterattacking with a barrage of almost unlimited legal resources. The lonely ombudsman enters a battle from which he or she will come out scarred and often deeply shaken, dealing with people who resist them and yet having to come back again and again and again. As one ombudsman put it, "when you go to a place where people block you, sabotage you, and refuse to talk to you how long can you take it?" One must look, however, at the other side of the coin, too. Mr. T. cautions: "Even sympathetic administrators of nursing home facilities feel affronted when their professional integrity and 20 or 25 years of experience are questioned by a newcomer who never set foot in a nursing home before." The state office of the ombudsman finds itself walking a tightrope: it has to back the volunteer technically and emotionally, otherwise the program will disintegrate, but it must not gratuitously offend the industry. "You have to convince them you are not out to destroy them, otherwise how can you return to them again the next day and the next week?"

Mr. T. observed that the very idea of operating with volunteers has turned into a political football with the nursing home industry:

> Initially they welcomed volunteers: they felt that the less training ombudsmen received, the less their capacity to make a dent in the system. They pictured volunteers as ineffectual nonentities who come and go. Now they are changing their tune: they want a professional ombudsman. Their argument that volunteers have few skills is correct, but this is only part of their strategy: they would like to have the program professionalized in order that ombudsmen can be better controlled. The industry is now convinced that a sure way of neutralizing the program is by making it part of the government's bureaucracy.

Mr. T. disagrees with the minimalist definition of the ombudsman role. He feels that their effectiveness is contingent on expanding rather than limiting their range of activities. He would like to see the program moving into policy analysis and quality control functions, including the opportunity to testify before the health systems agencies. These agencies are supposed to certify the need for new facilities and the expansion of the existing ones. If the ombudsman program of a given locality knows of repeated complaints or has valid reasons to doubt the quality of a conglomerate operating deficient homes elsewhere, it should be given the opportunity to testify to that effect to the health systems agencies. Mr. T. admitted that granting the ombudsman the right to testify will be tantamount to declaring war on the industry. "They will be out to crucify us."

Mr. T. also pointed out some of the philosophical and political dilemmas confronting the ombudsman program. When referring to an independent grass-roots organization for nursing home reform operating in two counties, he stated that "the industry is terrified of them and would like to squash them" but he also added that the social action group has little use for the ombudsman program because it finds it not aggressive enough and too identified with mediation, which in their opinion is sterile. "The ombudsman program is caught amidst the cross fire between the industry and the activists. The former label the ombudsmen volunteers as 'troublemakers.' The latter, in turn, accuse them of being 'patsies and collaborationists.' " The volunteers cannot help pondering about the meaning and actual reach of their neutrality. How much can they actually do against a powerful industry? If a home is found committing flagrant violations, the likelihood is that it will get away with a slap on the wrist. Is it in the interest of the ombudsman program to have the facility closed instead? "Where will the older residents be placed? They have nowhere to go."

The state ombudsman of an Eastern state also spelled out in unmistakable terms that ombudsmen have to operate beyond a supportive, therapeutic, and neutral framework. They are meant to be community advocates, not friendly visitors. An ombudsman, in her view, can be more of a confidant to the elderly residents than any staff member, but once that rapport has been established they have to proceed immediately to advocate for a solution. The drawback in the use of volunteers is that sometimes they accept complaints and voice problems too literally, relying on incorrect technical facts and lack of objectivity. In any event, friendly visitation can be legitimized as the initial phase in the advocacy process, but the program must remain committed to negotiating on behalf of the residents.

She dismissed the nursing home industry's contention that unless the volunteers are trained as full-fledged health professionals they are incapable of understanding the complexities of the long-term care delivery system. She saw no problem in the fact that volunteers are not versed in health matters. "It can allow them to be more representative and supportive of a patient who might otherwise feel alone and helpless. They are out there to advocate for a patient's better living conditions, not to understand all the technicalities of the services in place."

It was admitted that some volunteers do not have, in her words, "the guts to handle complaints." Therefore they prefer friendly listening. But that in itself is not a total loss because at least their presence makes the nursing home staff more responsive during those hours when they are present. Although it provides only minimum benefits, friendly visiting represents a real need for the institutionalized elderly, especially for those who have infrequent family visits.

> Friendly visiting creates the kind of atmosphere which allows them to reveal complaints. Many complaints, however, are handled by volunteers who simply do not report them in writing. Therefore it is as if the ombudsman volunteer does little more than friendly visiting, according to official reports.

This ombudsman added quite bluntly that "we would not need an ombudsman program if family and friends would act as advocates for patients." This highlighted the residual nature of the program as trying to make up for the lack of normal functioning of family and support networks. The goal that she spelled out is to have one volunteer for every fifty residents, an ideal yardstick since the program is far from reaching that goal. One county program pays its volunteers a stipend for the time they put in each week in the home. "This does not include the time necessary to travel to and from the nursing home nor extra time taken at home to write reports. But it does at least provide them a sense of recognition." She thinks that this mechanism of stipend provision has provided greater stability to the program and would recommend extending it to every county. The volunteers in this particular county are much more motivated, she finds. They seek additional training, are more "gutsy," and even have more of a sense of their own community. Another factor, perhaps, is that they set up a very good advisory committee and have close community backing. These two provisions together, the advisory committee and the stipend, seem to have facilitated a lot of success. However, much of it depends upon who is the head of the advisory committee and how that person can then proceed to utilize this mechanism to foster ombudsman program development.

Informants closely related to the ombudsman program were particularly sensitive to the factors and conditions that appeared to facilitate or, conversely, to inhibit the program's viability. The two surveys aimed to elicit information on the subject, but in a more structured way. The next section reports their findings.

Factors That Enhance or Hinder Program Effectiveness

The National Perspective

Ten items were measured in the national study as to the degree to which they constitute enhancing or restraining factors for the ombudsman program: funding levels, organizational placement of the ombudsman program, special interest group influence, state commissioners on aging, regional ombudsman training meetings, state office on aging staff, nursing home industry interests, legislative activities on long-term care, the governor's office, and citizens' organizations for nursing home reform. Respondents cautiously indicated that the vast majority of items were slightly enhancing of the ombudsman program. Major differences appeared, however, in the magnitude of such enhancements as perceived by the three major groups.

Both the aging interest group and the human services commissioners perceived nursing home industry interests as somewhat restraining of the ombudsman program—the only item to be identified as an inhibiting factor. The long-term care providers, on the other hand, viewed the item as somewhat positive. Analysis of variance revealed that the difference across groups was significant at p < .001. A similarly significant difference was indicated as to citizens organizations for nursing home reform. The aging interest group found this factor to be quite enhancing, the human services commissioners gave it moderate approval, and the long-term care providers perceived it to be of only slight importance.

Other items found to reflect significant differences included the regional ombudsman training meetings and legislative activities on long-term care. Both factors were seen as more enhancing by the aging interest group, but received lukewarm approval from the human services commissioners and the long-term care providers. State ombudsmen rated support from the commissioners on aging, Office on Aging staff, citizens' organizations, and from the governor's office equally as important in their enhancement ability as were links to legislative committees.

Foremost among the restraining factors was insufficient funding, supporting one former state ombudsman's characterization of the position as "almsbudsman." Resistance by the nursing home industry and the more general pressures of adversary interest groups were seen to be the next most serious restraints. The remaining factors—dealing with the organizational location of the state ombudsman program and relationships with the commissioner on aging and his/her staff—were seen as hardly serious impediments to programming at all.

A separate inquiry tapped the current organizational location of the state nursing home ombudsman program in all fifty states, Washington, D.C., and Puerto Rico. While almost one half of the state ombudsman programs are located in independent governmental units on aging, a third are situated within the governments' human service network—departments that may well have other procedural dealings with nursing homes, (such as licensing or reimbursement arrangements. This raises some question as to the presumed objectivity, independence, and impartiality that are imputed to the ombudsman in the literature. While about one in ten cases finds the ombudsman program under the aegis of the public executive, only two states reported that their nursing home ombudsman programs were contracted to private or voluntary organizations at the administrative level. Thus the trend is clearly toward the preference of governmental sponsorship in general, and in association with a state office on aging in particular, even if this sponsorship arrangement is at the expense of benefits accruing from an executive affiliation, or from a placement entirely outside governmental boundaries.

The New York City Perspective

Factors identified by community sponsors and professional program staff in New York City add depth to the review of those elements that affect program performance. Field interview data suggest four major locally relevant issues that warrant discussion.

First, consistent stress was placed on the program's lack of authority or clout. Repeatedly, agency representatives pointed to circumscribed staff powers and sanctions, lack of guaranteed access to facilities, negotiations primarily being carried out by "lower-level" staff, and a relatively weak link in the state government as inhibiting program success.

A second area of concern revolved around the use of volunteers. Difficulties in recruiting them, controlling the quality of the services they deliver, monitoring potential biases they may display, convincing them of the need for consistent and timely documentation of grievances, and instilling a clear understanding of the program's mission and function were factors most often voiced.

A third set of potential limitations centered on organizational capacity. It was felt by some that an inadequate number of professional staff, too loose and informal an administrative structure, and, in general, a lack of essential programmatic resources had become serious hindrances.

Finally, a number of field survey respondents were convinced that the program had not yet established proper linkages with voluntary community groups similarly concerned with quality care for the institutionalized aged.

Views from the Volunteers

Ombudsmen volunteers in New York City indicated that they were "fairly" to "very" satisfied with the experience of serving in the program. An additional measure of satisfaction was obtained when they were asked how long they intended to continue serving. Over half of those who responded to this question (52.2 percent) maintained they would be involved as long as the program is running, with an additional 21.7 percent prepared to serve for more than one year. The remaining ombudsmen indicated that they would not stay beyond their first year of service.

Over half again of volunteer ombudsmen indicated that serving in the program had changed the way they feel about older people and nursing homes. Among those whose opinions changed, the experience was somewhat more likely to have promoted negative views of the status of older people (53.3 percent) and conditions in nursing homes (53.3 percent) than positive perspectives.

Volunteers overwhelmingly pointed out that the most encouraging aspect of giving service had been the opportunity to put their altruistic impulses to concrete use, with a lesser number (31.0 percent) citing their sense of accomplishment as influencing their decision to remain with the program. Most prominent among the discouraging aspects of service that were cited was the feeling that their efforts lacked effect (46.4 percent) and the perceived insensitivity and lack of concern among long-term care staff (32.1 percent). Other disheartening aspects included the poor conditions in which the institutionalized aged lived (14.3 percent) and the amount of paper work the ombudsmen were required to complete (7.1 percent). Such data suggest an ambivalence between the volunteers' benevolent impulses and a sense of relative impotency when working within what appears to them as the intractable and rigid world of institutional life.

Value and Significance of the Ombudsman Program

Closely linked to an estimation of the ombudsman program's efficacy was the ultimate determination whether the program is altogether needed and whether its existence is justified. Members of the long-term care network, the group most directly challenged by the ombudsmen's presence, were asked to indicate the degree to which they agreed or disagreed with the following value statements:

1. The long-term care ombudsman program is a service which should be found in all long-term care facilities.
2. Most of the problems that the ombudsmen address would eventually be resolved by long-term care staff if ombudsmen were not there.
3. The long-term care ombudsman program fills a gap in the long-term care delivery system.
4. There is no real need for long-term care to be monitored by outside individuals or groups.
5. Even if outside regulatory agencies were fully able to ensure adequate care in long-term care facilities, ombudsman programs would still be needed.
6. The long-term care ombudsman program plays a unique role in the long-term care delivery system.
7. The long-term care ombudsman program unnecessarily duplicates the work of regulatory agencies that monitor long-term care.

Highly significant differences were obtained in analysis of variance across the three major groups of the national study on each of the value statements. Consistent response patterns were obtained as well. For each of the positive value statements (nos. 1, 3, 5, 6), the aging interest group showed a high degree of agreement, the human services commissioners a moderate one, and the long-term care providers indifference or a slight degree of disagreement. For each of the unfavorably worded value statements (nos. 2, 4, 7), as expected, the reverse trend was observed: the aging interest group showed strong disagreement, the human services commissioners a moderate degree of disagreement, and the long-term care providers only slight disagreement (no. 4) or moderate degrees of agreement (nos. 2 and 7).

The results clearly indicated, therefore, that the aging interest group is most convinced of the value of the ombudsman program, the human services commissioners guardedly assign only moderate value, and the long-term care providers have little use for it. When value perceptions were disaggregated by individual groups, comprising the respondent clusters, an identical trend, without deviation, was discerned. The results thus confirm the expression of a plurality of views, constituting a normative continuum along which the contribution of the ombudsman program toward assuring quality of long-term care is gauged.

Conclusion

The ombudsman is an external agent, alien to, yet inserted within, the fabric of nursing homes with a mission that the operators of these facilities rarely welcome. No wonder, then, that a series of effectiveness measures confirmed that the long-term care providers were the least convinced of the program's value. The aging interest group was, in turn, the most supportive of the ombudsmen's actions and *raison d'être*, while the human service commissioners placed themselves between these two polar positions with an ambivalent and often noncommittal attitude.

All respondent groups acknowledged, however, that the program realizes more favorable results when contending with matters of residents' rights and abuse. They also felt that the least effective areas were those of upgrading the nursing home staff and boarding homes' standards. The magnitude of intergroup effectiveness ratings differed significantly, however, with the aging interest respondent cluster granting, as usual, the highest, and the long-term care providers the lowest effectiveness ratings.

On facility level complaints, the identical response trend noted above emerged, but substantive differences were also discovered: human services commissioners and long-term care providers found the ombudsman program most effective on matters of food and nutrition in the facility, a complaint area to which the aging interest group assigned lesser importance. The latter granted, instead, higher program effectiveness in the area of health care, considered by human services commissioners to have been only moderately effectively coped with, and by the long-term care providers to have been least successfully approached. At the same time, all respondent groups were in agreement that the ombudsman program succeeded considerably in resolving problems inherent in the residents' interpersonal relations.

All respondents, and long-term care staff in particular, strongly associated mediative functions, and to a lesser extent therapeutically supportive behavior, with increased program effectiveness and impact. In the view of facility staff, the advocate function is not conducive to goal attainment. The volunteer ombudsmen perceived, in contrast, a broader range of program roles to be correlated with positive program performance. In essence, staff defined the ombudsman as a "specialist" in mediation, without conceding great significance to it. Ombudsmen saw themselves more as "generalists."

A final index of impact items corroborated trends observed throughout the study, but made the following distinction: long-term care providers viewed the greatest program influence in improving the quality of staff/resident relations in the nursing home, while other respondent groups thought they were only minimally affected. Conversely, the accountability of nursing home staff was viewed as most relatively affected by the aging interest group and the human services commissioners, but less so by their provider counterparts.

Data suggest that the advantages of utilizing volunteers rest on these individuals' high levels of altruistic concern for the institutionalized aged. However, these attributes may play against such obstacles to voluntary service provision as reduced time commitments, unbearable expenses, and limitations in acquired expertise.

A major finding is the relatively low visibility of the program among its intended beneficiaries. Grievances were considerably more likely to be voiced due to the initiative of the volunteer ombudsman than the institutionalized aged, and outreach efforts have least often served older females with limited education, receiving skilled nursing care and residing in facilities under proprietary auspice. Additional factors in ombudsman service usage were the resident population's fear of long-term care staff retaliation or else their inclination to deny the value of outside aid in the first place.

Overall, ombudsmen were judged to achieve moderate results. Most respondents felt that they do better in the interpersonal domain than in their efforts to bring about systemic policy-oriented changes. There were no outright expressions of rejection of the program's value. Whatever resistance staff had shown, it was mostly manifested as minimization or indifference, not as categorical opposition. All respondents also paid lip service to a normative if not experiential acceptance of the ombudsman's presence in nursing home facilities. The question of how to make this presence really work will be discussed in chapter 7.

CHAPTER SEVEN

The Future of the Ombudsman

What is the future outlook for the ombudsman program? What organizational and statutory supports are needed to make it work? Should it be continued?

In order to distinguish between varying outlooks concerning the preferred future of the nursing home ombudsman program, respondents in the national study were asked to rank the relative importance of several program resources. Two of the items—ombudsman-enabling legislation and mandated access to nursing homes'/patients' records—reflect necessary resources for an independent and residents' rights version of a long-term care quality assurance model. Conversely, the remaining item—a large indigenous volunteer pool—is an indicator of the kinds of resources needed for a more locally based and consensus-oriented, friendly visiting nursing home ombudsman program.

Differences in perceived importance of the three program resources were evident between the human services commissioners and the long-term care providers on the one hand, and the aging interest group on the other. The former saw the more general of the two residents' rights-focused resources—ombudsman-enabling legislation—as the most important of all the resources. On the other hand, mandated access, the more specific and rigorous of the rights-focused resources, was placed third in importance by the human services commissioners and by the long-term care providers.

The aging interest group, however, assigned an unqualified

first place ranking to mandated access to homes and records, presumably allowing for rights-focused inquiries by a nursing home ombudsman program. Enabling legislation followed in second place, with the remaining item assigned only tertiary importance. The aging interest group has clearly pointed to the rights-oriented resources as the most important for the ombudsman program while the other respondent groups adhere to these program resources with less conviction.

These trends are underlined by the findings of an analysis of variance. Significant intergroup mean differences were found on two of the three items in the ranking list. Mandated access, ranked first in importance by the aging interest group and only third by the others, yielded group mean differences significant at $p < .001$. Thus not only are the relative ranking differences noticeable, but the magnitude of assignments by each group is worthy of note as well. The aging interest group viewed this resource as more important than the human services commissioners, who in turn saw it as more important than the long-term care providers.

The question of needed resources was also broached from another perspective with similar results. Respondents were asked to indicate with which one of the following statements they most agreed:

1. Enabling legislation outweighs the importance of local program development.
2. Local program development outweighs the importance of enabling legislation.
3. Local program development is of equal importance to enabling legislation.

More than two thirds of the aging interest group found both program development and enabling legislation to be equally important, slightly less than two thirds of the human services commissioners did, and less than half of the long-term care providers. Long-term care providers tended to give more primacy to local program development than to enabling legislation and were significantly less ambivalent about the relative importance of enabling legislation and program development than the other two respondent groups. While a majority response did not emerge on the issue, data did reflect relatively greater long-term care provider insistence on the value of local program development to the detriment of enabling legislation.

The lack of support granted by long-term care providers to those resources that would facilitate a residents' rights approach was unmistakable. This and other differences of opinion among groups appear again in the data dealing with the preferred programmatic focus of the nursing home ombudsman program.

Preferred Program Focus

Activities

Respondents were asked to indicate their priorities for the following activities for future ombudsman programming:

1. Individual complaint resolution
2. Identification and publicity on issues in long-term care
3. Lobbying and legislative activity on behalf of long-term care
4. Community consumer education about long-term care alternatives
5. Citizen involvement in long-term care alternatives.

Due to observed differences among the original survey groups, respondents were not divided into the three analytic categories or major groups employed throughout the study. Rather, the responses of all eight respondent groups, including state nursing home ombudsmen, were analyzed.

Significant differences were manifested among respondent groups concerning the area of individual complaint resolution. Every group in the long-term care network ranked this activity as the most preferred of all future ombudsman program activities. In striking contrast, state ombudsmen, the principal actors who administer and spearhead program efforts, viewed individual complaint resolution as the least preferred of all five ombudsman program activities. Intergroup mean differences were significant at $p < .001$.

As noted earlier, the main rationale for instituting a "citizens' defender" for nursing home residents has traditionally been to provide appropriate redress for citizens' complaints. Furthermore, the initial activities of a state nursing home ombudsman program have typically been to elicit and address complaints of the institutionalized elderly. Members of the long-term care network perceive the program along those lines and prefer a continued individual complaint focus for the program in the future.

It would seem, however, that practical experience of the state nursing home ombudsmen has led them to the opposite conclusion. Repeated, and often futile, efforts to secure adequate redress for citizens' complaints have led them to advocate instead a range of supportive and/or preventive functions. They thus regarded the publicity of long-term care issues as the most important of future activities to be pursued. Second, they preferred developing a broader citizen involvement in long-term care. Again, experience has shown that many complaints are best handled by the continuous on-site monitoring and negotiation that locally based volunteers can best carry out. Hence issue publicity and citizen involvement take precedence in the eyes of the ombudsmen, paving the way to more successful resolution of individual complaints of nursing home residents. Interestingly, these two areas also obtained significant group mean differences in the statistical analysis. Publicity of long-term care issues was ranked the second most preferred activity by most respondent groups, but fourth by proprietary nursing home associations and last by citizen advocacy organizations. Conversely, citizen involvement was ranked second by these latter two groups along with the state ombudsmen, but considered a very low priority by the remainder of respondents. Group differences on these two items were significant at p < .01. The remaining two activity areas, lobbying and consumer education, were given middle to low priority by all respondent groups as future ombudsman program activity priority areas.

Overall findings suggest major differences in view between the deliverers of ombudsman services for the aged in long-term care, and the long-term care organizational network, in the preferred future activity of patient representation. In order to determine whether preferred future activity differed significantly from current ombudsman program activity, statistical comparisons were made for each program item, for both "current" and "future" rankings. Findings confirm that ombudsmen assigned significantly lower priority to individual complaint resolution in the future. Commissioners on aging and welfare similarly preferred less focus on the future handling of individual complaints. While not achieving statistical significance in the differences between current and preferred future activity rankings, none of the remaining respondent groups wished to see more attention placed upon individual complaint resolution than is presently given.

Significant differences between current perceptions and preferred future focus upon publicity of issues in long-term care were found for only one group: the proprietary nursing home associations. Needless to say, they wished to see such publicity substantially reduced in the future.

In turn, the ombudsmen's front-line experience lead them to deemphasize individual complaint resolution, a wish shared by commissioners on aging and welfare, and to stress greater citizen involvement. Legal services developers and citizens' advocacy organizations also supported greater citizen involvement as the major change in the program. Commissioners of health and welfare indicated higher priority on education for long-term care alternatives. The not-for-profit nursing home associations were unable to commit themselves to a particular desired program change, thus reflecting their lack of familiarity with the ombudsman program. Finally, the proprietary nursing home associations desired less publicity on issues, and greater consumer education and citizen involvement in long-term care, presumably as friendly visitors.

Organizational Placement and Accountability

The question of optimal placement for a nursing home ombudsman program, within or outside governmental control, has been debated among ombudsman program planners and ombudsmen themselves. Remaining within the halls of public office provides opportunities for access to officials and administrative advocacy that would not otherwise be possible. Placement outside government, on the other hand, enables ombudsmen greater freedom to pursue legislative and litigative advocacy on behalf of nursing home residents.

Which administrative location is the most preferred in terms of program effectiveness and accountability? Respondents were asked to indicate their preferred placement for promoting optimal ombudsman program effectiveness: office on aging, governor's office, department of health or social service, or private organizations.

Two trends were discerned. First, most respondents preferred a governmental as opposed to a nongovernmental placement. The aging interest group expressed the greatest inclination for the latter, but even so that choice accounted for only a quarter of the respondents from that group. Second, a majority, as in the case of the aging interest group, and a plurality, as in the other two major groups' responses, preferred placement in the state office on aging. This location, it may be suggested, provides the greatest potential for an independent ombudsman program within government.

Interestingly, of all the major respondent groups, the greatest support for placing the ombudsman program in the governor's office was expressed by the long-term care providers. Given this group's limited appreciation of the program, and differing preferences regarding its future role and focus, it is plausible to surmise that such placement would provide a more direct avenue for influence by long-term care providers on ombudsman programming.

Statutory Empowerment

The last of the prescriptive areas surveyed was the extent of statutory powers desirable for an ombudsman program. It may be recalled from the review of the literature in chapter 1 that statutory regulation has been a major characteristic of classical ombudsmen. Statutory empowerment has traditionally been interpreted to imply the capacity to investigate and make recommendations but not the power to revise or reverse administrative action. Recent applications of the ombudsman concept, on the other hand, have seen the ombudsman function expand its acquisition of statutory powers to a greater range of tasks. It is most relevant, therefore, to examine the positions of the three major groups on this matter.

Respondents were presented with a list of five variations of statutory power, and asked to indicate how important they are for the functioning of an ombudsman program. The kinds of powers rated included:

1. Statutory authority to change decisions made in nursing homes
2. Statutory authority to enforce decisions made in nursing homes
3. Mandated access to all nursing homes
4. Mandated access to all patient records
5. Legislative/legal authority in performing their functions.

Power items 1 through 4 represent specific measures of program power whereas power item 5 is viewed as a generalized measure. Tests of internal scale consistency confirmed high reliability for the instrument both for the New York City study ($\alpha = .86$) and the national survey ($\alpha = .85$). Internal correlation coefficients between all power items ranged from .34 to .83 in the local survey and .38 to .90 for the national investigation.

A review of the scale findings revealed strong consistency with the major trends identified earlier in the study. Each power item was viewed as most needed by the aging interest group, second most needed by the human services commissioners, and least important by the long-term care providers. Internal rankings indicated identical ordering within each group, but the magnitude of the differences across groups strongly overshadowed this apparent congruence in the pattern of response.

Absolute scores showed that the aging interest group strongly supported mandated access to facilities and to patients' records, and the granting of legal authority for the ombudsman function. Their view that ombudsmen should be given the statutory right to change or enforce decisions made in nursing homes, on the other hand, was less emphatic but still somewhat favorable. The human services commissioners expressed recognition of the importance for mandated access to nursing homes and legal authority to perform the ombudsman function, but only slight importance for access to patient records. Conversely, they indicated some disagreement as to the importance of statutory authority to change or enforce decisions made in nursing homes.

The long-term care providers expressed clear opposition to the overall statutory empowerment of the nursing home ombudsman program as indicated both by item scores and by the composite power measure. While they allowed a guarded recognition of support for access to nursing homes and a semblance of legal authority for the ombudsman, they somewhat opposed access to patients' records and strongly rejected any formalized authority aimed at neutralizing internal decisions made by nursing homes.

Findings obtained in the New York City study paralleled, to a large extent, those of the national survey. Volunteer ombudsmen expressed the greatest need for additional program powers. Their views were quite similar to those of their advisory board members who were slightly less emphatic about additional program powers. In sharp contrast with these views, the three categories of long-term care staff—administration, directors of nursing, and directors of social services—were in close agreement that the ombudsman program should not be given more legal authority. The minimal concern voiced by long-term care staff for enlarged program authority was consistent with their rejection of the suggestion that ombudsmen should assume an advocate role. When long-term care staff were disaggregated by institutional auspice, proprietary staff gave significantly less support to the idea of power enlargement than did staff working in voluntary facilities.

Positive correlations were found among volunteer ombudsmen and long-term care staff between perceived need for power acquisition and importance assigned to the advocate role. This correlation reached a level of significance in the case of the ombudsmen and approached signifiance in the case of long-term care staff. For the latter the need for program power tends to be negatively correlated with the mediator role and the therapeutic role, though these findings were not statistically significant. A negative correlation between power acquisition and both the mediator and the therapeutic support roles did not appear in the case of the volunteer ombudsman. It would seem that the volunteers do not rule out the need for additional power merely because they subscribe to less political, nonpartisan ombudsman roles. Acquiring more power may be considered beneficial in their efforts at performing a range of interventive tasks.

Ombudsmen also interpreted that patients see them as having more power/authority than they actually command. While patients' data did not directly address this aspect of the power issue, other findings supported the ombudsmen's emphasis on the need for additional program authority. Thus, among those institutionalized respondents who maintained that they knew about the ombudsman program, 55.3 percent agreed that they did not think the volunteer ombudsman had enough authority to solve nursing home problems. It may be that the perceived "inflated" views of the individual ombudsman's authority felt to be held by residents served as additional stimulus for the volunteers seeking greater program leverage within the institution.

The differences emerging from both the national and the New York City studies encompass varying prescriptions for the structure and function of the nursing home ombudsman program. The implications of these findings for program planning will be considered in the next section on a normative model for long-term care ombudsman services.

A Normative Model of Nursing Home Ombudsman Services

When considered together, the quantitative survey findings, observational data from on-site field visits, and nursing home ombudsman program reports collected for the two studies point to an ombudsman program development process valid for most state nursing home ombudsman programs. Furthermore, findings clarify major points of divergence in the implementation of this program development process. The choices inherent in ombudsman program development, and the rules that govern their selection, portend significantly varying outcomes for the structure and function of ombudsman services for the institutionalized elderly.

A typical pathway in the development of a state nursing home ombudsman program is sketched in the following scenario. While variations are to be found in many states, the process outlined here constitutes an "ideal type" of construction, against which individual state ombudsman programs may be compared.

The state nursing home ombudsman program begins with major emphasis placed on the establishment of a complaint processing mechanism, similar to the classical origins of the ombudsman function. Unlike the classical ombudsman, however, the initial nursing home ombudsman program functions without the legislative sanction associated with its classical counterpart. The absence of legislative support and the exigencies of program development move the ombudsman program to seek first to regularize its staffing and funding patterns.

The program is initially staffed by a single government employee who seeks cooperation from associates in state government, and particularly in state units on aging. As the program gets under way, constrained by limited funding, the state ombudsman moves to recruit volunteers to carry out program functions. The eventual provision of funding regularity, however, as required by the 1978 amendments to the Older Americans Act, has allowed as well for expansion of salaried central staff, contracting with local public or private organizations in complaint elicitation and the subsidization of some volunteer activity.

Thus in its initial phase, the state nursing home ombudsman program, composed of a single ombudsman, engages in simultaneous visitation of nursing homes and verification of complaints as well as in program development and resource acquisition. With basic funding assured, the state ombudsman moves from being service-oriented to becoming a development specialist. Focus shifts from direct complaint handling to building ombudsman program capacity, and accordingly to expansion of program coverage across the state.

When local, or substate, units of a state nursing home ombudsman program come into being, a search for program identity and role clarity among local ombudsman volunteers commences. The roles of facility watchdog, impartial mediator, and friendly visitor are tested to varying degrees, and responses from facility staff, residents, and the community at large are gauged. Essential resources required for the fulfillment of these respective roles are identified and attempts are made to recruit them. Role conflict from within and opposition external to the ombudsman program become manifest. Efforts are made to clarify differential state and local ombudsman functions.

The role and function of the state level ombudsman program become crystallized, expressed in the recruitment and training of regional salaried staff who will in turn put local and area program initiatives into operation. The state ombudsman, furthermore, engages in efforts to formulate and to gain passage of enabling legislation from state government and to ensure legitimation and functional regularization of the ombudsman program at all levels. Concurrently, the state ombudsman works to develop and formalize channels of cooperation with other organizational components of state government, particularly those that regulate aspects of long-term care. Efforts at interorganizational cooperation extend simultaneously to relevant voluntary associations of long-term care providers and grass-roots citizens' groups to broaden the program's support.

The local-level ombudsman programs, on the other hand, concentrate upon identifying, recruiting, and maintaining a volunteer pool. Individual ombudsman volunteers are assigned to visit long-term care facilities and to engage in the identification, investigation, and resolution of residents' complaints. The focus is more often than not on a consensually oriented exchange between ombudsman program personnel and the operators of the long-term care facility.

If enabling legislation has not yet been enacted, the local program turns toward a focus on maximizing its coverage of facilities, and reaching greater numbers of aged residents in long-stay institutions. At the same time, the program initiates efforts to publicize its function. Publications are distributed, posters hung, and mass media sources tapped. Once the local program is firmly established, its main focus turns to handling the complaints received from the residents of the area nursing homes.

With local-level ombudsman programs in place, the function of the state's nursing home ombudsman programs become two-pronged. Local-level projects handle residents' complaints and attempt to resolve them within the facility, through consensual strategies and mutual agreement. Complaints that involve infractions of rights or legal codes and severe abuse are referred to appropriate regulatory agencies in the state government. Statistics reflective of the nature and frequency of complaints are identified, gathered, and forwarded on a monthly basis to the state ombudsman.

The state ombudsman subsequently engages in systematic compilation of complaint statistics across the state. Trends are identified and common problems or issues isolated. The focus then turns to issue advocacy in which the state ombudsman, with the help of the state unit on aging and state-level citizens' groups, communicates long-term care issues to the public. Legislative action is advocated for in the case of those issues evidencing greatest severity and frequency of occurrence. Inroads are also sought in preventing the emergence of complaints stemming from discovered gaps or inadequacies in the delivery system of long-term care.

The evolution of the state nursing home ombudsman program can thus be traced through a process in which initial efforts to establish a state-level complaint mechanism give way to program function at state and local levels. Local ombudsman volunteers, under the supervision of paid regional and area staff, engage in individual advocacy on behalf of nursing home residents. Their activities, when adequately documented, free the state ombudsman in turn to engage in issues advocacy on a larger scale.

Overview of Study Findings

The preceding discussion highlights the formative phases of a hypothetical program and abstracts the most common state experiences. Before drawing together the program implications of this research, it is useful to review its major conclusions.

Chapters on study findings characterized state ombudsmen as balancing their time across a range of activities, including program development, individual complaint advocacy, and issue advocacy. These professionals, it may be recalled, were heavily invested in drawing public support and encouraging the organization of local programs. They also took the lead in the recruitment, training, and placement of the volunteer participants. State ombudsmen were thus doing many things at one and the same time. Such plurality of program foci reflected, on occasions, a sound and premeditated planning course. On others, it was an accommodation to adverse political circumstances. Ombudsmen frequently found themselves engaged in an uphill quest for identity and survival.

Volunteers who staff the local programs were primarily recruited due to their own altruistic motivation or desire to help. Once recruited, however, their continued participation largely required technical support mechanisms such as staff training and supervision. Monetary stipends played a minor role in the initial recruitment or retention of volunteer participation, but may be of symbolic value as a means of reinforcing volunteer activity.

Citizens' organizations and grass-roots advocacy groups have been involved with the nursing home ombudsman program largely in a back-up capacity. State ombudsmen drew their organizational support, rather, from governmental service and regulatory agencies, with which they maintained the most frequent contact. Furthermore, the staff of the offices on aging, and particularly commissioners on aging, were seen to offer the ombudsman program the greatest degree of organizational support.

On the negative side, federal efforts to supply regional training and the sharing of information among state ombudsmen were disregarded by state ombudsmen as effective enhancements to program efforts. Long-term care provider associations were seen to have the least frequent contact, and assign the least value for the planning and provision of ombudsman services for the institutionalized elderly.

Inquiry into problem focus of the ombudsman program suggested that the areas most frequently addressed (residents' rights, abuse of residents, and consumer education for long-term care) were accordingly considered the least difficult to resolve. Problems less frequently addressed, on the other hand, such as relocation trauma, residents' participation in policy-setting, and Medicaid discrimination, were seen to be both more difficult to cope with and resolve.

Among facility complaints, nutrition (food quality) was the area most frequently dealt with by the ombudsman program, and concurrently the most resolvable. Conversely, other frequently handled complaints (those related to health care, protection of personal property, administration, and personal care) were seen as those most impervious to redress.

Comparisons between state and local levels of the ombudsman program function revealed that proposing policy changes and providing information for legislators and planners were most effectively carried out at the state level. Conversely, state ombudsmen maintained that local-level efforts were significantly more effective in alerting facility staff to patients' needs. Similarly, state ombudsmen found that substate programs realize significantly greater impact on improving nursing home/community and staff/residents relations. Long-term care facility staff accountability, on the other hand, was seen to be equally affected by both the state and local levels of the ombudsman program.

Findings thus suggested that areas related to the establishment and enforcement of patient rights were most effectively dealt with at the state level. The day-to-day operations of the long-term care facility that affect the quality of life, on the other hand, were seen to be most successfully addressed by the mediational intervention of a local-level ombudsman program.

The long-term care network presented a range of perceptions of, and responses to, the nursing home ombudsman program, identifiable for three major categories of respondents: the aging interest group maintains the most frequent contact with the ombudsman program; the long-term care providers indicate the least frequent contact with the ombudsman program, and similarly impute the least value to such contact; human services commissioners fall between the other two groups in their perceptions of both frequency and value of contact with the ombudsman program. The aging interest group was most convinced of the value of the ombudsman program, the human services commissioners guardedly assigned only moderate value, and long-term care providers saw little value at all for this program in assuring quality of care.

Divergent responses across the three groupings were upheld in considering the accuracy of a range of ombudsman role descriptions and evaluations of efficacy. While all respondents tended to favor the mediational roles of middleman, listener, and guide, the accuracy of these roles as descriptions of ombudsman behavior differed markedly across the respondent groups. Of particular note was the reluctance of long-term care providers to define any role as accurately reflecting local ombudsman activity. Provider associations appear either resistant to legitimatizing ombudsmen functions or unaware of exactly how the local ombudsman mandate is being carried out. The aging interest group was markedly distinguishable from both the human services commissioners and the long-term care providers in its high rating levels concerning the program's effectiveness and impact. The findings indicate that those not identified *a priori* as an interest group on behalf of the elderly are still far from acknowledging the nursing home ombudsman program's positive attributes. Furthermore, evidence suggests that perceptions of ombudsman program function and performance may be heavily influenced by one's own affiliation and normative stance in the long-term care system.

Looking toward a future scenario for the nursing home ombudsman program, the aging interest group clearly preferred those program resources that allow for an advocacy-oriented ombudsman service (mandated access to nursing homes). Long-term care providers, on the other hand, granted little legitimacy to those resources that would facilitate a residents' rights approach.

In regard to roles that the local ombudsman may occupy, the aging interest group preferred adversarial roles to the collaboratively geared therapeutic role model favored by long-term care providers. Human services commissioners were divided on this question, with commissioners of health for a contest-motivated therapeutic role for the ombudsman. Interestingly, state ombudsmen themselves identified a collaborative-based brokerage role for the local level ombudsman.

When considering future program foci, long-term care providers were distinguishable from other respondents in their preference for a developmental focus that emphasizes the need to target upon the nursing home resident. Human service commissioners favored a watchdogging focus with the resident in mind. The aging interest group, on the other hand, preferred watchdogging, but with a focus on nursing home facility issues.

This succinct overview points to conflicting perceptions about the program's accomplishments and disparate positions concerning its ultimate *raison d'être*. This is to be expected, given the multiplicity of actors involved. They range from government agencies to human rights organizations, networks of grass-roots and national organizations on behalf of the aged, institutionalized, long-term care patients, and a privately owned and voluntary, not-for-profit, long-term care service industry. Last but not least, there are the community volunteers. They are the central characters, the heroes—or the villains—of this story, depending on whose viewpoint is being considered. Most would agree that the role the volunteer ombudsmen take on is a risky one, fraught with uncertainty and exceeding their limited repertoire of technical competence.

The study exposed the public stance of each of the actors. By scrutinizing their ideological premises it also hinted at their hidden agendas. It is a truism to comment that each has a different stake in the program's continuance. Some would retain its secondary expressive features as a symbolic concession only, but would neutralize any semblance of formal authority. Others see its effectiveness contingent on an enlargement of the ombudsman's statutory right to intervene. Wavering between the two are those who would legitimize the less confrontational aspects of the role and assimilate it into the battery of therapeutic interventions already practiced by other professions. They surmise that institutions would then feel less threatened by the intrusive volunteers, and would then tacitly acquiesce to broadening their role.

Some ombudsmen and their sponsors think that such accommodation is feasible. Others view it as tantamount to its emasculation and ultimate destruction. In any event, when juxtaposing the descriptive scenario of the preceding section and the study findings, two divergent paths emerge: the two routes the ombudsman program may pursue to ensure its survival.

Program Development Pathways and Recommendations

Rules which govern the progression of an ombudsman program through one or another development path are many and complex. This section identifies the components of each program development pathway, and some of the criteria that influence choice.

Chart 7.1 presents in summary fashion the range of relevant program dimensions investigated in this study, and their respective characteristic features in each of the two potential program models. It should be noted that the dimensions and characteristics are dichotomized as exclusive "ideal types" for the sake of analytic comparison. In all likelihood, however, each dimension constitutes a continuum of choice for which the respective program pathway components serve as end points. Thus a given state nursing home ombudsman program may be placed at any point on the continuum for each program dimension. The reasons for placing a given program at one rather than another point along the continua are considered subsequent to presentation of the pathway models.

As can be seen from this chart, state nursing home ombudsman programs may develop along the path of a patients' rights program model, or the path of a quality-of-life-oriented model, each with its concomitant set of programmatic characteristics. Sets of such components are grouped within three dimen-

Chart 7.1
Program Development Pathways

Ombudsman Program Dimension	Program Development Path 1	Program Development Path 2
BASIC PHILOSOPHY		
Goal/mission	Patients' rights	Quality of life
Operational objectives	Watchdogging protective regulations	Providing emotional and developmental support
Advocacy focus	Issue/system	Individual
View of target groups	Consumers/citizens	Clients/patients
Interventive orientation	Adversarial/partisan	Collaborative/supportive
EXTERNAL ORGANIZATIONAL ISSUES		
Sanction/mandate	Statutory empowerment	Informal cooperation
Organizational placement	Government-based	Voluntary organization
Interorganizational linkages	Formal	Informal
Funding source	Legislation	Grass-roots fundraising
Scope	Statewide	Facility-focused
INTERNAL MANAGEMENT ISSUES		
Staffing pattern	Salaried	Volunteer
Recruitment strategies	Professional outreach	Altruistic motivation
Training foci	Stress on advocacy skills	Stress on therapeutic skills
Retention mechanism	Coalition with legal services/citizens' organizations	Intensive supervision
Administration	Autonomous	Supervisory
Publicity	Mass media	Networking
Accountability	Compilation of complaint statistics	Group-oriented communication in supervision
Record-keeping	Standard legal forms	Expressive narratives

sions. basic philosophy, external organizational issues, and internal management issues.

A summary statement of the patients' rights model sees this form of ombudsman program as a statutorily empowered, government-based program, statewide in scope and formalistic in its organizational relations, that has been established and funded through state legislation. The basic approach of the patients' rights model entails a watchdogging focus, partisan on behalf of long-term care consumers and geared toward systemic changes. Such programs are staffed by professionals, specialists in legal and long-term care regulatory matters, who engage in joint efforts with public interest law representatives and citizens' organizations. The patients' rights ombudsman utilizes complaint statistics compiled through formal record-keeping to advocate for policy changes that will positively impact upon those areas of recurring complaints.

The qualify-of-life program model, on the other hand, is more often than not an informal consortium of voluntary organizations which work through their own fund-raising efforts and gain informal bases of cooperation at the long-term care facility level. The basic approach of this model may be said to be a collaborative one in which volunteers work with facility personnel to support individual nursing home patients who have expressed some difficulty. Such volunteers are recruited through their own strong desire to aid others, and are sustained by peer support and intensive supervision from local ombudsman program support staff. The focus of the quality-of-life ombudsman is the improvement of the day-to-day life of nursing home patients by ameliorating interpersonal conflict with facility staff, or with other patients.

What determines whether a given nursing home ombudsman program will (a) develop in the predominant direction of one pathway or the other, (b) select a varied mix of components from each path model, or (c) attempt the simultaneous operationalization of both models for ombudsman services? Clearly, there is no single formula to predict a specific outcome for a developing nursing home ombudsman program. Variations can be seen to occur due to the degree of financial and legislative resources made available to the evolving ombudsman service, the scope of the necessary coverage, and other factors that may or may not be influential in a particular state. A selected list of such factors that shape decision rules and which in turn determine program choices follows. Additional factors invariably should be identified for each state engaged in ombudsman program development. The factors identified in this study include:

1. The funding level and/or presence of alternative sources of financial support
2. The size of the institutionalized aged population
3. The scope and configuration of the long-term care system
4. The influence of special interest groups
5. The status of enabling legislation
6. The status of alternative state regulatory and monitoring systems
7. Community norms/public attitudes
8. Predilections of the state's chief executive
9. The history of past abuse in long-term care
10. The demography of the state's elderly population (size, ethnicity, and rural/urban composition).

Based upon this study's findings, it is suggested that ombudsman programs should seek to be more responsive to locally relevant criteria. Lack of fit may jeopardize effectiveness and impact. The two program pathways outlined in Chart 7.1 are equally legitimate courses to follow. It may be that local programming will more easily take on the characteristics of Path 2 and state-level efforts those of Path 1. Nevertheless, conditions may dictate the appropriateness of one strategy or the other, regardless of geographic scope.

While a single ombudsman program may exhibit elements borrowed from both developmental pathways, as this mix of program dimensions increases so will organizational complexity and the potential blurring of roles and functions. Programs need to be aware of the implications of such a mix and guide their operations accordingly. Decisions will need to be made in such situations as to whether specialists in advocacy and collaboration are preferable to generalists capable of operating in both domains.

It is therefore conceivable that programs may follow both orientations to ombudsman programming at certain points, depending on the types of grievances elicited. In that case it may be useful to maintain ongoing lines of communication with ombudsman operating within both pathways to facilitate consultation on unusual situations that demand alternative orientations.

Finally, there may be particular program elements that will fare poorly together, such as informal cooperation as a sanction and a patients' rights focus, or lack of mesh between training foci and basic philosophy. Training program curricula need to be reconsidered in light of the models which have been offered. Specialized training curricula responsive to varying program orientations will then be required.

Implementation of either program path presupposes that a policy and planning framework as well as a set of organizational resources have already been set in place. However, research findings provide abundant evidence that such conditions are, for the most part, still evolving in what often appears to be a painstaking trial-and-error process. The following recommendations are not prescriptive formulas for program success. They are intended, however, to lessen the risk factor in program development and accelerate its incrementalistic course. Moreover, these recommendations are a synthesis of comments elicited from all survey respondents, coupled with analysis of secondary data sources. Their selection obviously reflects the authors' own judgments and inevitable biases.

1. POLICY

a) Legislation needs to consolidate the right of access to all levels of institutional care. Ombudsmen should not be prevented from entering any long-term care facility or approach the patients residing there.

b) Legislation should provide incentives for various modes of primary group and voluntaristic involvement (families, relatives, community groups) in institutional life, to counter the tendency toward excessive organizational rigidity and formalization.

c) Administrative sanction should be given at the local level to independent, voluntary sponsors with a community-wide and balanced scope of interest. Central state authority should be retained in the office of the governor with formally defined linkages to all human and health services departments.

d) Legislation should give greater recognition to the broad range of role behaviors that have evolved in the provision of ombudsman services, including the mediative, advocacy, and therapeutic approaches. Statutory guides to program development ought to reflect a more eclectic and flexible stance rather than a doctrinaire adherence to a classical formula of program action.

e) Legislative action is needed to foster the planning and ultimate implementation of centralized data collection on patient abuse and neglect. This effort should be coordinated with the development of a national long-term health care data set.

f) National legislation needs to be sharpened and focused to better ensure that each state will operate an effective ombudsman network. Current policy provisions allow too great a range in effort, from exemplary undertakings to programs that are little more than "paper tigers."

g) Support is needed for greater levels of information sharing among state programs. States should exchange information on effective interventive procedures and reflect the positive inputs and interests of all pertinent professional and interest groups.

2. PROGRAMMING

a) Programs should encompass personal advocacy functions as well as an orientation to systemic and broader policy change requirements.

b) Volunteer ombudsmen programs should underscore a generalist orientation to local practice, with more specialized back-up resources provided by professional staff. Such an arrangement will capitalize on the altruistic perspective of the volunteer while attending to high service standards.

c) Ombudsman programs should resolve potential conflict due to overlapping functions with long-term care facilities staff. Dysfunctional and potentially duplicative efforts should be carefully monitored and resolved through negotiation.

d) Community advisory boards are needed at the local level to ensure genuine sponsorship from all concerned parties. They should include adequate representation by long-term care administrators and other facility personnel, community agency professionals, residents and their families, and the interested general public.

e) Volunteer ombudsman programs need to stress continuity and consistency of effort. Regularized rather than erratic visits to facilities will build trust, increased visibility, and clarity of program function. Continuity should be linked to intensified outreach efforts aimed at the older, less educated, and female residents, most especially in proprietary facilities.

f) Training of volunteer ombudsmen needs to be refined and enriched in the understanding that ombudsmen are frontliners and that they are not intended to substitute for the professional staff. They could still benefit from greater degrees of preparation in the areas of investigative skills, entitlements, licensing codes, negotiation methods, and bargaining.

g) Programs should provide opportunities for volunteer advancement. The more capable and dedicated volunteers should be assigned supervisory and training responsibilities, and given the option to negotiate with external community support networks.

h) The stress and potential discouragement that may accompany the work in long-term care facilities highlight the importance of a range of incentives continuously available to the ombudsman volunteer. They include rotating placements, a stipend program, peer support groups, opportunities for advancement on a volunteer career ladder, and attendance at skills development training workshops and conferences.

3. RESEARCH

a) Systematic evaluation efforts should begin as close to program inception as possible.

b) Time-series designs and longitudinal research may best determine whether ombudsman services are able to bring about changes in grievance resolution rates, reductions in the manifestation of particular types of problems, decreases in complaint recidivism rates, and increases in the level of satisfaction among residents/patients with their conditions of life.

c) Research may also focus on the differences of impact of services on both nonprofessional and professional long-term care staff and seek to gauge the perceptions of friends and relatives of the institutionalized aged.

d) Research continues to be needed in the area of the relative efficacy of utilizing volunteers versus salaried personnel and possible variation in the rates of program success in rural and urban settings.

e) Finally, studies should assess the impact of selected ombudsman sociodemographic characteristics (age, sex, professional background, ethnicity) on their role behavior and functional orientation.

EPILOGUE

The value of the long-term care ombudsman concept lies in the possibility that it may bridge the individual needs of the institutionalized aged with general systems reform. Volunteer ombudsmen, unencumbered by routine organizational structures, have already given proof of considerable in-depth involvement with the problems of the most vulnerable elderly. Their program is the only line of defense for many citizens living in closed environments and ordinarily lacking effective recourse over decisions affecting their lives.

It makes no sense, however, to stereotype staff and administrators of nursing homes as perennial scapegoats. Many of their decisions are judicious and compassionate. Others seen as arbitrary may well be the inevitable corollary of a high-pressured environment where workers must respond to a myriad of institutional crises all at once. The merits of such decisions and practices may be, however, less of an issue than the fact that they cannot be challenged. It is the absence of readily available mechanisms of appeal and redress that the elderly often find humiliating. Patients' rights, nominally embodied in existing statutes, are not worth the paper they are printed on unless provisions are concurrently made to ensure their enforcement. Ombudsmen are placed in the long-term care system precisely to oversee the proper respect for those rights. Their job is to enable residents to express grievances whenever they feel victimized. It does not take much for people who always led independent lives and are now suddenly confined to a regimented institution to feel helpless and in despair. By restoring a measure of self-determination to their lives, the ombudsman may be countering those negative feelings. The consensual versus adversarial goal dichotomy discussed throughout this book may be less real than it seems. Restoring people's sense of control over their destiny has implicit therapeutic consequences whether obtained through mediation or advocacy.

It is this personalized approach to service delivery which distinguishes ombudsman program effort from that of other quality assurance mechanisms. Regulators, prosecutors, and legal agents, although invested with considerably more authority, lack the capacity—and the mandate—to maintain close person-to-person connections with their clients at all times. The ombudsman's sensitivity to patients' needs, coupled with the direct and immediate feedback they provide, is its mark of distinction. In essence, the efficacy of institutional ombudsmen may be largely determined by their capacity to maintain an individualized focus on the one hand and a "worldly-wise" appreciation for systemic remedies on the other. It is still too early to judge whether this balancing of perspectives is attainable, and above all, whether it can endure.

In any event, the program has realized measurable success in selected areas. It proved capable of introducing advocacy and mediating strategies, among others, into many closed long-term care institutions, a feat not to be lightly dismissed. The major test, however, is yet to come. It may be contained in the recently proposed reduction in enforcement provisions for federal nursing home regulations. Ombudsmen will find their job far more difficult if the already minimal standards presiding over the long-term care system are to be weakened. It is quite possible that the statutory mandate of the ombudsman program may be nullified and swept away in the wake of the process started with President Reagan's Executive Order requiring the reduction or elimination of burdensome regulations (Executive Order #12291, February 17, 1982). It is not inconceivable, either, that the ombudsman program's short-lived legacy will then be to arouse a "second generation" of volunteers to come to the defense of the institutionalized elderly. Their strategies and auspices may be different. They may not even call themselves ombudsmen and they may blend with current citizens' rights groups for nursing home reform. Their sense of mission will be, however, just the same.

Whatever its future format or sponsorship, the ombudsman idea will remain a valid indicator of society's concern for its most vulnerable citizens, while having to accept the reality of long-term care institutions in its midst.

APPENDIX A
SCALE CONSTRUCTION AND RELIABILITY TESTING

Appendix A contains information on each major scale constructed for both the New York City and national studies. Information provided includes the number of items included in each scale, the identities of those items, the obtained reliability coefficients, and the range in metric ratings for individual items.

1. *ROLE PERCEPTION SCALE* (*New York City and National*)
    Item 1.   Making easier the conditions of residents
    Item 2.   Guiding the residents through the proper channels
    Item 3.   Serving as a middleman between the nursing home and the residents
    Item 4.   Arguing the cause of the residents
    Item 5.   Serving as an impartial listener
    Item 6.   Translating the rules and regulations of nursing home residents
    Item 7.   Explaining decisions of others to residents
    Item 8.   Observing staff practices in nursing homes
    Item 9.   Reforming and improving staff practices in nursing homes
    Item 10. Occupying a watchdogging position to insure adequate nursing home conditions
    Item 11. Providing emotional support to residents/patients

            Reliability coefficient (NYC)   = .88
            Reliability coefficient (national) = .91

Potential scale-item range: 1–5, where 1 = very accurate role and
                              5 = not very accurate role at all

Respondent groups: New York City and state ombudsmen
                     New York City advisory board members
                     New York City long-term care staff
                     State long-term care network

2. *PROGRAM POWER SCALE (New York City and National)*
   Item 1.   Statutory authority to change decisions made in nurs-
             ing homes
   Item 2.   Statutory authority to enforce decisions made in nurs-
             ing homes
   Item 3.   Mandated access to all nursing homes
   Item 4.   Mandated access to patient records
   Item 5.   Legislative/legal authority in performing their function

              Reliability coefficient (NYC)   = .86
              Reliability coefficient (national) = .85

Potential scale-item range:
   For New York City study items 1, 2, 3, and 4: 1–5, where 1 = very
      important power and 5 = not important power
   For New York City study item 5: 1–2, where 1 = important power
      and 2 = not important power
Potential scale item range for national study:
   1–5, where 1 = very important power and 5 = not important
      power

Respondent groups: New York City and state ombudsmen
                     New York City advisory board members
                     New York City long-term care staff
                     State long-term care network

3. *EXPERIENCED EFFECTIVENESS SCALE (New York City)*
   Item 1.   Sensitive to your concerns
   Item 2.   Respectful to you
   Item 3.   Interested in your problem
   Item 4.   Competent to deal with your problem

Item 5.   Able to keep you informed about the results of the attempts to solve your problem

Reliability coefficient (NYC) = .91

Potential scale-item range: 1–5, where 1 = strongly agree and 5 = strongly disagree

Respondent group: New York City nursing home patients

4. *PERCEIVED EFFECTIVENESS SCALE (New York City)*
Item 1.   Assist in the protection of patients' rights
Item 2.   Establish a speedy mechanism for resolving residents' complaints
Item 3.   Propose changes in nursing home policies and regulations
Item 4.   Increase communication among nursing home staff and residents
Item 5.   Establish better relationships between community and nursing home groups
Item 6.   Improve the day-to-day life of long-term care residents
Item 7.   Provide information for legislators and program planners for bringing about changes in long-term care
Item 8.   Prevent the recurrence of service deficiencies in long-term care facilities
Item 9.   Alert nursing home staff and administration to patients' needs
Item 10. Support changes in nursing home policies and regulations

Reliability coefficient (NYC) = .88

Potential scale-item range: 1–5, where 1 = not successful at all and 5 = extremely successful

Respondent groups: New York City ombudsmen
New York City advisory board members
New York City long-term care staff

5. *PERCEIVED EFFECTIVENESS SCALE* (*National*)
Item 1. Propose changes in nursing home policies and regulations
Item 2. Establish better relationships between community and nursing home groups
Item 3. Provide information for legislators and program planners for bringing about changes in long-term care
Item 4. Establish a speedy mechanism for resolving resident complaints
Item 5. Assist in the protection of patients' rights
Item 6. Alert nursing home staff and administration to patients' needs
Item 7. Develop a statewide ombudsman network
Item 8. Develop an information clearinghouse
Item 9. Provide public education on long-term care

Reliability coefficient (national) = .92

Potential scale-item range: 1–5, where 1 = not successful at all and 5 = extremely successful

Respondent groups: State ombudsmen
                     State long-term care network

6. *PERCEIVED IMPACT SCALE* (*New York City*)
Item 1. The severity of problems in nursing homes
Item 2. The general quality of services in facilities
Item 3. The accountability of staff actions in nursing homes
Item 4. The degree of patient/resident participation in decisions affecting their lives
Item 5. The quality of nursing home/community relations
Item 6. The quality of relations among staff in nursing homes
Item 7. The satisfaction of residents with services received in the facility
Item 8. The overall social climate within nursing homes
Item 9. The quality of staff/residents relations in nursing homes

Reliability coefficient (NYC) = .81

Potential scale-item range: 1–9, where 1 = very negative effect and 9 = very positive effect

Respondent groups: New York City ombudsmen
                      New York City advisory board members
                      New York City long-term care staff

7. *PERCEIVED IMPACT SCALE (National)*
    Item 1.   The accountability of staff actions in nursing homes
    Item 2.   The quality of nursing home/community relations
    Item 3.   The quality of relations among staff in nursing homes
    Item 4.   The quality of staff/residents relations in nursing homes

              Reliability coefficient (national) = .81

Potential scale-item range: 1–5, where 1 = very negative effect and
                               5 = very positive effect.

Respondent groups: State ombudsmen
                      State long-term care network

8. *ISSUE EFFECTIVENESS SCALE (National)*
    Item 1.   Residents' rights
    Item 2.   Abuse of residents
    Item 3.   Nursing home regulations/enforcement
    Item 4.   Medicaid discrimination
    Item 5.   Upgrading nursing home staff
    Item 6.   Relocation trauma
    Item 7.   Boarding home standards (adult homes, RCF's)
    Item 8.   Consumer education relating to long-term care
    Item 9.   Alternatives to institutionalization in long-term care fa-
              cilities
    Item 10. Mental health needs of long-term care facility residents
    Item 11. Abuse of residents' funds
    Item 12. Residents' participation in facility governance

              Reliability coefficient (national) = .92

Potential scale-item range: 1–5, where 1 = not effective at all and
                               5 = extremely effective

Respondent groups: State ombudsmen
                      State long-term care network

9. *COMPLAINT EFFECTIVENESS SCALE* (*National*)
   Item 1. Food/nutrition
   Item 2. Administration
   Item 3. Environmental safety
   Item 4. Facility sanitation
   Item 5. Interpersonal relations (residents)
   Item 6. Personal care (help with washing, dressing)
   Item 7. Health care
   Item 8. Personal allowance
   Item 9. Protection of personal property

Reliability coefficient (national) = .94

Potential scale item range: 1–5, where 1 = not effective at all and
                              5 = extremely effective

Respondent groups: State ombudsmen
                     State long-term care network

APPENDIX B
SCALE DIMENSION
VALIDATION

A ten-member expert panel, composed of social welfare experts throughout New York State and Connecticut, was asked to rate various New York City study variables as to their degree of fit along eight proposed subscale dimensions. Degree of fit could potentially range from a high of 1 to a low of 7.*
The eight proposed dimensions were meant to tap major components of ombudsman role behavior, program effectiveness, and program impact as postulated by the researchers. The panel was first asked to familiarize themselves with the dimensional definitions offered and then to proceed to rate the extent of fit of each role, effectiveness, and impact item included in the questionnaires. Three potential dimensions of role behavior (mediator, advocate, and therapeutic support), three potential dimensions of program effectiveness (policy/planning, organizational/programmatic and relationship/interac-

---

*An example of the procedure:
Ex. *Social Science Dimension:* A dimension including all social science disciplines

Discipline		*Degree of Fit*					
	HI						LO
1. Sociology	x						
	1	2	3	4	5	6	7
2. Physics							x
	1	2	3	4	5	6	7
3. Anthropology			x				
	1	2	3	4	5	6	7

tive), and two potential dimensions of program impact (technical service and social) were presented to the panel as defined below:

I. *ROLE BEHAVIOR*
   1. *MEDIATOR DIMENSION*
      This dimension includes those factors that stress nonpartisan roles taken in relating to different individuals or groups of individuals. These factors should be free of bias, nonjudgmental, and intermediary in nature.
   2. *ADVOCATE DIMENSION*
      This dimension includes factors that stress active partisan roles taken in relating to different individuals or groups of individuals. It encompasses the pleading or defending of the rights of others.
   3. *THERAPEUTIC SUPPORT DIMENSION*
      This dimension includes those factors that serve to promote social adjustment or heightened personal well-being and comfort among individuals or groups of individuals.
II. *PROGRAM EFFECTIVENESS*
   4. *POLICY/PLANNING DIMENSION*
      This dimension includes those factors that relate to structural changes within a system that are broad or systemic in nature, having collective rather than individual consequences.
   5. *ORGANIZATIONAL/PROGRAMMATIC DIMENSION*
      This dimension includes those factors that deal with specific operating program processes within particular settings having consequences for individuals or groups of individuals.
   6. *RELATIONSHIP/INTERACTIVE DIMENSION*
      This dimension includes those factors that encompass interpersonal or socializing aspects of program activity. These are qualitative in nature, centering on exchanges between individuals or groups of individuals.
III. *PROGRAM IMPACT*
   7. *TECHNICAL SERVICE DIMENSION*
      This dimension includes those factors that relate to program and organizational functions in a particular setting. These activities are seen to impinge on the lives of individuals or groups of individuals.

8. *SOCIAL DIMENSION*
   This dimension includes those factors that focus on interactions of a qualitative nature between individuals or groups of individuals, within or outside a particular setting.

The three lists of factors (role, effectiveness, and impact items) whose degree of fit was judged within each corresponding set of dimensions are in Appendix A.

The Student-Neuman-Keuls Procedure was used to identify ranges in panel ratings for the p <.05 level. It allowed for the identification of homogeneous subsets for factor items and ultimately validated the assignment of seven of the original eleven role behavior items to the three proposed role behavior dimensions, three of the original ten program effectiveness items to two proposed effectiveness dimensions, and four of the original nine program impact items to the two proposed impact dimensions. The items composing each dimension are:

1. *ROLE PERCEPTION SCALE DIMENSIONS*
   Mediator Dimension
      Role Item 3: Serving as a middleman between the nursing home and residents
      Role Item 7: Explaining decisions of others to residents
   Advocate Dimension
      Role Item 4: Arguing the cause of the residents
      Role Item 9: Reforming and improving staff practices in nursing homes
      Role Item 10: Occupying a watchdog position to ensure adequate nursing home conditions
   Therapeutic Support Dimension
      Role Item 1: Making easier the conditions of residents
      Role Item 11: Providing emotional support to residents/patients

2. *PERCEIVED EFFECTIVENESS SCALE DIMENSIONS*
   Policy/Planning Dimension
      Effectiveness Item 3: Propose changes in nursing home policies and regulations

Effectiveness Item 7: Provide information for legislators and program planners for bringing about changes in long term care

Relationship/Interactive Dimension

Effectiveness Item 5: Establish better relationships between community and nursing home groups

3. *PERCEIVED IMPACT SCALE DIMENSIONS*

Technical Impact Dimension

Impact Item 3: The accountability of staff actions in nursing homes

Social Impact Dimension

Impact Item 5: The quality of nursing home/community relations

Impact Item 6: The quality of relations among staff in nursing homes

Impact Item 9: The quality of staff/residents relations in nursing homes

NOTES

Introduction

1. The Federal Council on the Aging, "The Need for Long Term Care," p. 2.

2. U.S. Department of Commerce, Bureau of the Census, *Current Population Reports, Special Studies; Siegal, Demographic Aspects of Aging and the Older Population in the United States.*

3. National Center for Health Statistics, "Current Estimates from the Health Interview Survey, United States, 1978."

4. The Federal Council on the Aging, "The Need for Long Term Care," p. 30.

5. National Center for Health Statistics and Hing, "Nursing Home Residents."

6. Moss and Halmandaris, *Too Old, Too Sick, Too Bad.*

7. Weatherby, "Regulation of Nursing Homes," p. 309.

8. Regan, "When Nursing Home Patients Complain, pp. 695–96.

9. Vladeck, *Unloving Care.*

10. Henry, *Culture Against Man.*

11. Kayser-Jones, *Old, Alone and Neglected.*

12. Bennett, "The Meaning of Institutional Life," pp. 117–25; Pincus, "Toward a Conceptual Framework for Studying Institutional Environments in Homes for the Aged"; Kosberg and Tobin, "Variability Among Nursing Homes," pp. 214–29.

13. Coe, "Self Conception and Institutionalization," pp. 225–53; Lieberman, Tobin, and Slover, "The Effects of Relocation on Long Term Geriatric Patients."

14. Stannard, "Old Folks and Dirty Work," pp. 329–42; Blumenthal et al., *Justifying Violence.*

15. Kayser-Jones, *Old, Alone, and Neglected,* p. 7.

16. Sullivan, *Corrective Mechanisms for Resolving Abuses and Upgrading Care in Institutions for the Aged.*

17. Donabedian, "Evaluating the Quality of Medical Care," pp. 166–70; New York State Moreland Act Commission, *Regulating Nursing Home Care;*

Weatherby, "Regulation of Nursing Homes," p. 309; Regan, "When Nursing Home Patients Complain," pp. 695–96.

18. Anderson, "Developing the Ombudsman Role in Health Care Services," pp. 1–5.

19. Regan, "When Nursing Home Patients Complain," pp. 695–96.

20. Donabedian, "Evaluating the Quality of Medical Care," pp. 166–70.

21. Regan, "Quality Assurance Systems in Nursing Homes," p. 53.

22. Weatherby, "Regulation of Nursing Homes," p. 309.

23. Wildavsky, *Speaking Truth to Power*, pp. 288–89.

24. Decker and Bonner, eds., *PSRO*, p. 7; Gosfield, *PSRO's*, p. 16.

25. Gosfield, p. 16; Vladeck, *Unloving Care*, p. 169.

26. Vladeck, p. 169; *ibid.*, p. 170.

27. Decker and Bonner, eds., *PSRO*, p. 45.

28. Forman, "The Nursing Home Ombudsman Demonstration Program," pp. 128–33.

29. Regan, "Quality Assurance Systems in Nursing Homes," p. 53.

30. *Ibid.*

31. Delany and Davies, *Nursing Home Ombudsman Project Final Report.*

32. U.S. Government, *Federal Register.*

33. Barney, "Community Presence as a Key to Quality of Life in Nursing Homes," pp. 265–68.

34. Gottesman and Gourestom, "Why Nursing Homes Do What They Do," pp. 501–6.

35. Eggert et al., "Caring for the Patient with Long Term Disability," pp. 102–18.

36. Moss and Halmandaris, *Too Old, Too Sick, Too Bad.*

1. Antecedents of the Ombudsman Program

1. Rowat, *The Ombudsman*, and Gellhorn, *Ombudsmen and Others.*

2. Ascher, "The Grievance Man or Ombudsmania," p. 175.

3. *Ibid.*

4. Broderick, "One-legged Ombudsman in a Mental Hospital," p. 522.

5. Verkuil, "The Ombudsman and the Limits of the Adversary System," p. 846.

6. Regan, "When Nursing Home Patients Complain," pp. 695–696.

7. Rowat, *The Ombudsman*, p. 8.

8. Appearing in *The Ombudsman: Citizen's Defender*, 2d ed. (1968), p. xxiv.

9. Gellhorn, *Ombudsmen and Others*, pp. 420–39.

10. Hill, "The New Zealand Ombudsman's Authority System," and "Institutionalization, the Ombudsman, and Bureaucracy"; *Ombudsmen, Bureaucracy, and Democracy*, p. 1077.

11. Northey, "New Zealand's Parliamentary Commissioner," in Rowat, *The Ombudsman*, p. 127.

12. Hill, "Institutionalization, the Ombudsman, and Bureaucracy," p. 1077.

13. Moore, "Ombudsman and the Ghetto," p. 246.

14. Gwyn, "The British PCA," pp. 50, 56.

15. Stacey, *Ombudsmen Compared.*

16. Dolan, "Pseudo-Ombudsman," pp. 297–301.

17. In Sandler, "An Ombudsman for the United States," p. 105.

18. Gellhorn, *Ombudsmen and Others,* p. 192; Linnane, *Ombudsman for Nursing Homes.*

19. Wyner, ed., *Executive Ombudsmen in the United States,* p. 10.

20. Anderson, "Comparing Classical and Executive Ombudsmen," in *ibid.*

21. Wyner, ed., *Executive Ombudsmen in the United States,* pp. 11, 10.

22. Hill, "Institutionalization, the Ombudsman and Bureaucracy," pp. 1076–77; Wyner, ed., *Executive Ombudsmen in the United States,* p. 312; Penn, "Advocate from Within."

23. Gwyn, *Barriers to Establishing Urban Ombudsmen,* p. 67.

24. Regan, "When Nursing Home Patients Complain," p. 666; Wyner, ed., *Executive Ombudsmen in the United States,* p. 311.

25. Fitzharris, *The Desirability of a Correctional Ombudsman,* p. 57.

26. *Ibid.,* pp. 58, 59; Gellhorn, *Ombudsmen and Others.*

27. Stacey, *Ombudsmen Compared.*

28. Tibbles, "Ombudsman for American Prisons," pp. 426, 427.

29. Cromwell, "A Vote for the Jail Ombudsman," pp. 54–56.

30. Williams, "Between the Keepers and the Kept," pp. 33–36.

31. Fitzharris, *The Desirability of a Correctional Ombudsman.*

32. Anderson, Moore, and Cressey, "The Prison Ombudsman," pp. 6–10.

33. *Ibid.*

34. *Ibid.*

35. Fitzharris, *The Desirability of a Correctional Ombudsman,* p. 69.

36. Williams, "The Minnesota Corrections Ombudsman," pp. 6–10.

37. Stewart, "What a University Ombudsman Does," pp. 1–29.

38. Verkuil, "The Ombudsman and the Limits of the Adversary System," p. 850.

39. *Ibid.,* p. 861.

40. Silverbank, "Role Perceptions of the Ombudsman," pp. 238–39.

41. Grafton and Rivera, "Student Perceptions of the Ombudsman's Role in a Community College," pp. 365–68; also see, for example, Adams, "School Ombudsmen Explore Student Rights," pp. 24–27; Larson, *Ed-Om.*

42. Stewart, "What a University Ombudsman Does," pp. 1–29.

43. Harvey, "Comment on What a University Ombudsman Does."

44. *Ibid.*

45. Laking, "The Ombudsman and Medicine," p. 412.

46. *Ibid.*

47. Kopolow, "Meeting the Patients' Rights Challenge through Mental Health Advocacy," p. 384; Madison, "Those Who Speak Up," p. 30.

48. Broderick, "One-legged Ombudsman in a Mental Hospital, p. 526.

49. Katz, "Advocacy in a Total Institution," pp. 215–16; Ettlinger, "Advocate Informs Patients of Rights and Responsibilities," p. 465.

50. Robb et al., "Advocacy for the Aged." pp. 1737–38; Abrams, "A Contrary View of the Nurse as Patient Advocate," p. 262.

51. Katz, "Advocacy in a Total Institution, p. 215; Kopolow, "Meeting the Patients' Rights Challenge through Mental Health Advocacy," p. 383; Madison, "Those Who Speak Up," p. 30; Robinson and Alboim, "The Use of Non-professional Change Agents in an Institution," pp. 469–72.

52. Eckert, "Advocacy in the Context of the Sociology of Knowledge."

53. Mailick, "Patient Representative Programs in Short Term General Hospitals and Their Relation to Social Work."

54. Wolkon and Moriwaki, "The Ombudsman," pp. 229–38.

55. Payne, "Ombudsman Roles for Social Workers," p. 99.

56. Zweig, "The Social Worker as Legislative Ombudsman," p. 26.

57. Fox, "The Ombudsman," pp. 50–51.

58. Hazard, "The Ombudsman."

59. Cloward, "An Ombudsman for Whom?" pp. 117–18; and Cloward and Elman, "Poverty, Injustice and the Welfare State: Part 1," pp. 230–35.

60. Payne, "Ombudsman Roles for Social Workers," p. 98.

61. Mallory, "The Ombudsman in a Residential Institution," pp. 14–17; Felton et al., "New Roles for New Professional Mental Health Workers," pp. 53–54; Pletcher, "The Curriculum Ombudsman," pp. 73–75.

62. Battle, "The Role of the Pediatrician as Ombudsman in the Health Care of the Young Handicapped Child," pp. 916–22; Koltveit, "Counselor-Consultant as Quasi-Ombudsman," pp. 198–200; Nelson and Starck, "The Newspaper Ombudsman as Viewed by the Rest of the Staff," pp. 453–57.

63. Smith and Winnick, "Your Library," pp. 6–11; Park and Shapiro, "Being Your Child's Ombudsman at School and Elsewhere," pp. 29–32; Milliken and Urich, "The Community Ombudsman," pp. 59–62.

64. For a more detailed discussion of advocacy functions see Grosser, "Community Development Programs Serving the Urban Poor"; Brager, "Advocacy and Political Behavior"; Davidoff, "Advocacy and Pluralism in Planning"; Grosser, "A Polemic on Advocacy"; McGowan, *Case Advocacy.*

65. Grosser, "Community Development Programs Serving the Urban Poor."

66. Grosser, *New Directions in Community Organization,* p. 276.

67. Gilbert and Specht, "Advocacy and Professional Ethics," p. 288; Berger, "An Orienting Perspective on Advocacy"; Annas and Healey, "The Patient Rights Advocate, p. 258; Wolfensberger et al., *The Principle of Normalization in Human Services.*

68. Annas and Healey, "The Patient Rights Advocate," p. 258; Payne, "Ombudsman Roles for Social Workers," p. 98; Moore, "Ombudsman and the Ghetto," p. 245; Mallory, "The Ombudsman in a Residential Institution," p. 15.

69. Broderick, "One-legged Ombudsman in a Mental Hospital," p. 524; Regan, "When Nursing Home Patients Complain," p. 708.

70. Verkuil, "The Ombudsman and the Limits of the Adversary System," pp. 846, 851.

71. Broderick, "One-legged Ombudsman in a Mental Hospital," p. 562; see also Lowi, The End of Liberalism.

72. Annas and Healey, "The Patient Rights Advocate," p. 259; Moore, "Ombudsman and the Ghetto," p. 261.

73. Mallory, "The Ombudsman in a Residential Institution," p. 16; Sosin, "Social Work Advocacy and the Implementation of Legal Mandates," pp. 265–73.

74. Regan, "When Nursing Home Patients Complain," p. 735.

75. Ibid., pp. 737–38.

2. Structuring Quality Assurance Mechanisms for the Elderly in Long-Term Care

1. Luke and Boss, "Barriers Limiting the Implementation of Quality Assurance Programs," p. 305. For a range of positions on the subject see, for example: Brody, Long Term Care of Older People; Kahana, "Matching Environments to Needs of the Aged," pp. 210–14; Kosberg, "Making Institutions Accountable," pp. 510–16; and Pincus and Wood, "Methodological Issues in Measuring the Environment in Institutions for the Aged and Its Impact on Residents," pp. 117–26.

2. Donabedian, The Definition of Quality and Approaches to Its Assessment.

3. Luke and Boss list a range of assurance strategies, such as the bicycle approach, the tracer method, health accounting, and the quality assurance monitor. They note "the appropriate strategy in quality assurance is unclear and depends upon such factors as the level and type of care provided, the resources or information base, and the purpose of the assessment" (Luke and Boss, "Barriers Limiting the Implementation of Quality Assurance Programs," pp. 305–6).

4. Gustafson et al., "Measuring the Quality of Care in Nursing Homes," pp. 336–43; and Howard and Strong, "Evaluating the Quality of Nursing Home Care," pp. 525–26.

5. Anderson, "Approaches to Improving the Quality of Long Term Care for Older Persons," pp. 519–24, identifies two criteria useful in evaluating the quality of care: patient outcomes and accessibility of the facility to the community. Linn, Gurel, and Linn, "Patient Outcomes as a Measure of Quality of Nursing Home Care," pp. 337–44, similarly view patient outcomes of survival and discharge to be positively associated with service provision (R.N. hours per resident and high meal service ratings); Kahn et al., "A Multidisciplinary Approach to Assessing the Quality of Care in Long Term Care Facilities," pp. 61–65, point out the limitations of medical diagnoses as indicators of quality care since such diagnoses alone do not reflect

the unmet needs of long-term care residents. George, *Quality of Care in Nursing Homes*, cites the difficulty of providing quality care in nursing homes due to high turnover and low morale among the nonprofessional staff; and finally, Stannard, "Old Folks and Dirty Work," pp. 329–41, notes the invisibility of patient/aide interaction which creates the potential for patient abuse and prevents the effective assurance of quality care.

6. Chapuisat, "Le Mediateur Français ou l'Ombudsman Sacrifié," p. 109.

7. Hill, *The Model Ombudsman*, p. 248.

8. Nancoo, "Administrative Theory and Bureaucratic Control," p. 246.

9. Hill, *The Model Ombudsman*, p. 14.

10. Danet, "Toward a Method to Evaluate the Ombudsman Role," p. 363.

11. *Ibid.*

12. Friedmann, "The Public and the Ombudsman," p. 498.

13. Burbridge, "Problems of Transferring the Ombudsman Plan," p. 105.

14. Danet and Hartman, "Coping with Bureaucracy," pp. 7–22.

15. Friedmann, "The Public and the Ombudsman," p. 522.

16. Anderson, "The Ombud and Health Services," pp. 89, 97.

17. Laking, "The Ombudsman and Medicine," p. 412.

18. Anderson, "Developing the Ombudsman Role in Health Care Services."

19. Anderson, "The Ombud and Health Services," pp. 97–98.

20. *Ibid.*, p. 99.

21. Pugh, "On Being an Ombudsman."

22. Anderson, "The Ombud and Health Services," p. 100.

23. *Ibid.*, p. 101.   24. *Ibid.*, p. 92.   25. *Ibid.*, p. 103.   26. *Ibid.*, p. 104.

27. Love and Rechnitzer, "Patient Rights and the Elderly," p. 3.

28. Wilson, "Nursing Home Patients Rights," p. 261.

29. Daley and Jost, "The Nursing Home Reform Act of 1979," pp. 448–54.

30. Caldwell and Kapp, "The Rights of Nursing Home Patients: Possibilities and Limitations of Federal Regulation," p. 44.

31. *Ibid.*, pp. 46–47.

32. Loeser et al., "Federal Regulation of Medical Practice in Nursing Homes," pp. 512–14.

33. National Citizens' Coalition for Nursing Home Reform, "A Report on the White House Mini-Conference on the Rights of the Institutionalized Elderly and the Role of the Volunteer," p. 2. For further legislative developments, see National Citizens' Coalition for Nursing Home Reform, "A Report on 1980 State Nursing Home Legislation," and National Citizens' Coalition for Nursing Home Reform, "State Nursing Home Legislative Update."

34. Sosin, "Social Work Advocacy and the Implementation of Legal Mandates."

35. Etzioni, "The Third Sector and Domestic Missions," p. 322.
36. Berger and Neuhaus, *To Empower People,* p. 6.
37. Langton, ed., *Citizen Participation in America.*
38. Jordan, "Voluntarism in America," p. 495.
39. O'Connell, "From Service to Advocacy to Empowerment," p. 198.
40. Adams, *On Being Human Religiously,* p. 81.
41. Langton, "The New Voluntarism," p. 10.
42. *Ibid.,* p. 15.
43. Vosburgh, "Client Rights, Advocacy and Volunteerism," p. 43.
44. *Ibid.,* p. 44.
45. Vosburgh and Hyman, "Advocacy and Bureaucracy."
46. *Ibid.*
47. Reeder, "The Patient-Client as Consumer," pp. 406–12.
48. Huttmann, *The Patient's Advocate,* p. 203.
49. Haug, "Doctor Patient Relationships and the Older Patient."
50. Parsons, "The Sick Role and the Role of the Physician Reconsidered," pp. 276–77.
51. Freidson, "Dominant Professions, Bureaucracy and Client Services," p. 441.
52. See, for example, Ferguson and Tydeman, "Organizing Around Nursing Home Issues," and Tydeman, "Putting the Pieces Together."
53. For a look at how the consumerist approach is put into operation in a state-wide nursing home ombudsman program see Citizens for Better Care and Anson, *Organizer's Manual for Nursing Home Ombudsmen.*
54. Haug, "Doctor Patient Relationships and the Older Patient," p. 859.
55. *Ibid.*
56. Neugarten, "The Future and the Young-Old," pp. 4–9.
57. Sundram, "Independent Oversight of Mental Hygiene Facilities," p. 45.
58. *Ibid.,* pp. 45–46.
59. New York State Commission on Quality of Care for the Mentally Disabled, "Boards of Visitors," p. 7.
60. Sundram, "Independent Oversight of Mental Hygiene Facilities, p. 46.
61. Cohen, "The English Board of Visitors," p. 24.
62. *Ibid.,* p. 27.
63. The development of the Florida Long Term Care Ombudsman Committee is chronicled in a series of annual reports published by the state of Florida. *Annual Report of the Nursing Home Ombudsman Committee.*
64. See Pateman, *Participation and Democratic Theory.*
65. Shore, "Try a Residents' Council," p. 140.
66. Silverstone, *Establishing Resident Councils,* p. 8.
67. Shore, "Try a Residents' Council," p. 139.
68. *Ibid.*

69. See Silverstone, "Expert Vs. Consumer Viewpoints: An Organizational Analysis of the Contrasts in Descriptions of Homes for the Aged by Administrators and Indigenous Residents."

70. See King County Coalition of Nursing Home Resident Councils, *The Bulletin.*

71. Newmark, "The Development of a Residents' Council in a Home for the Aged," p. 22.

72. *Ibid.*, p. 24.

73. Shore, "Try a Residents' Council," p. 140.

74. Parker and Shields, *Resident Council Resource Kit,* p. 2.

75. Kauffman and Boyle, "Family Advisory Councils in the Long Term Care Facility," pp. 51–60.

76. See, for example, Sullivan, *Corrective Mechanisms for Resolving Abuses and Upgrading Care in Institutions for the Aged,* especially ch. 2, and Clarke, "Communicating with Residents and Their Families," pp. 11–17.

77. Trueblood and Anderson, "Nursing Home Ombudsmen Involvement with Resident Governance in Homes for the Aging," p. 1.

3. Study Methodology

1. Strahan, "Inpatient Health Facilities Statistics, United States, 1978."

4. The Ombudsman and the Complaint Grievance Process

1. State of Connecticut, "An Act Creating a Nursing Home Ombudsman Office."

2. Connecticut Nursing Home Ombudsman Office, "Annual Report."

3. *Ibid.*, p. 5.

4. Fay, "Annual Report of the Ombudsman for the Institutionalized Elderly."

5. *Ibid.*, p. 4.   6. *Ibid.*, p. 4.

7. State of Florida, the Adult Congregate Living Facilities Act of 1975, ch. 75–233 as amended by ch. 77–401, as reported in State of Florida, "Annual Report of the Nursing Home Ombudsman Committee," p. 1.

8. *Ibid.*, p. 94.   9. *Ibid.*, p. 93.   10. *Ibid.*, p. 1.

11. State of Florida, "Annual Report of the Long Term Care Ombudsman Committee," p. 89.

12. "Older Americans Advocacy Assistance Program," pp. 1–3.

13. Massachusetts Department of Elder Affairs, "Massachusetts Older Americans Advocacy Assistance Program Semi-Annual Report," p. 14.

14. Citizens for Better Care and Anson, *Organizer's Manual for Nursing Home Ombudsmen,* p. i.

15. *Ibid.*, Preface, p. i.   16. *Ibid.*

17. Nursing Home Interests Staff, Administration on Aging, "The Nursing Home Ombudsman Demonstration Program," p. 20.
18. *Ibid.*
19. Hunter, "A Plan for a New York State Nursing Home Patient Ombudsman Program."
20. New York State Office for the Aging, Nursing Home Patient Ombudsman Program, "New York State Office for the Aging Nursing Home Patient Ombudsman Program, First Annual Report, 10/1/77–9/30/78."
21. *Ibid.*, pp. 27–28.
22. New York City Nursing Home Patient Ombudsman Program, "Outline of Nursing Home Patient Ombudsman Program Interaction with Long Term Care Facilities," p. 1.
23. State of Florida, "Annual Report of the Long Term Care Ombudsman Committee," p. 86.

5. What Do Ombudsmen Do?

1. Felton et al., "New Roles for New Professional Mental Health Workers," pp. 53–54.
2. Mailick, "Patient Representative Programs in Short Term Hospitals and Their Relation to Social Work."
3. Regan, "When Nursing Home Patients Complain," pp. 737–38.
4. Nursing Home Interests Section, Administration on Aging, "The Nursing Home Ombudsman Demonstration Program."
5. Forman, "The Nursing Home Ombudsman Demonstration Program."
6. Linnane, *Ombudsman for Nursing Homes.*

6. Do Ombudsman Programs Get Results?

1. New York City Nursing Home Patient Ombudsman Program, *OmbudsNews,* pp. 1–2.

BIBLIOGRAPHY

Abrams, Natalie. "A Contrary View of the Nurse as Patient Advocate." *Nursing Forum* (1978), vol. 17, no. 3.

Adams, James Luther. *On Being Human Religiously.* Boston: Beacon Press, 1976.

Adams, John K. "School Ombudsmen Explore Student Rights." *Opportunity* (April 1972), vol. 2, no. 3.

Anderson, Nancy N. "Approaches to Improving the Quality of Long-Term Care for Older Persons." *The Gerontologist* (December 1974), vol. 14, no. 6.

Anderson, Stanley V. "Comparing Classical and Executive Ombudsmen." In Alan J. Wyner, ed., *Executive Ombudsmen in the United States.* Berkeley: Institute of Governmental Studies, University of California, 1973.

—— "Developing the Ombudsman Role in Health Care Services." *Public Affairs Report* (June 1974), vol. 1, no. 3.

—— "The Ombud and Health Services." *Journal of Health and Human Resources Administration* (August 1979), vol. 2, no. 1.

Anderson, Stanley, John Moore, and Donald Cressey. "The Prison Ombudsman." *The Center Magazine* (November 1975).

Annas, George J. and Joseph M. Healey. "The Patient Rights Advocate: Redefining the Doctor-Patient Relationship in the Hospital Context." *Vanderbilt Law Review* (March 1974), vol. 27, no. 2.

Ascher, Charles S. "The Grievance Man or Ombudsmania." *Public Administration Review* (June 1967), vol. 27, no. 2.

Barney, Jane. "Community Presence as a Key to Quality of Life in Nursing Homes." *American Journal of Public Health* (March 1974), vol. 64, no. 3.

Battle, Constance. "The Role of the Pediatrician as Ombudsman in the Health Care of the Young Handicapped Child." *Pediatrics* (December 1972), vol. 50, no. 6.

Bennett, Ruth. "The Meaning of Institutional Life." *The Gerontologist* (September 1963), vol. 3, no. 3 (Part 1).

Berger, M. "An Orienting Perspective on Advocacy." In Paul A. Kerschner, ed., *Advocacy and Aging*. Los Angeles: University of Southern California Press, 1976.

Berger, Peter and Richard John Neuhaus. *To Empower People*. Washington, D.C.: American Enterprise Institute for Public Policy Research, 1977.

Blumenthal, Monica D. et al. *Justifying Violence*. Ann Arbor: Institute for Social Research, University of Michigan, 1971.

Brager, George. "Advocacy and Political Behavior." *Social Work* (April 1968), vol. 13, no. 2.

Broderick, Albert. "A One-Legged Ombudsman in a Mental Hospital: An Over-the-Shoulder Glance at an Experimental Project." *Catholic University Law Review* (Spring 1973), vol. 22, no. 3.

Brody, Elaine M. *Long Term Care of Older People: A Practical Guide*. New York: Human Sciences Press, 1977.

Caldwell, Janice M. and Marshall B. Kapp. "The Rights of Nursing Home Patients: Possibilities and Limitations of Federal Regulation." *Journal of Health Politics, Policy and Law* (Spring 1981), vol. 6, no. 1.

Chapuisat, Louis-Jérôme. "Le Mediateur Français ou l'Ombudsman Sacrifié." *International Review of Administrative Sciences* (April–June 1974), vol. 40, no. 2.

Citizens for Better Care and Robert E. Anson, Jr. *Organizer's Manual for Nursing Home Ombudsmen*. Detroit: Citizens for Better Care, 1976.

Clarke, T. R. "Communicating with Residents and Their Families." In *Proceedings of the Fifth North American Symposium on Long Term Care Administration*. Washington, D.C.: American College of Nursing Home Administrators, 1976.

Cloward, Richard. "An Ombudsman for Whom?" *Social Work* (April 1967), vol. 12, no. 2.

Cloward, Richard and Richard Elman. "Poverty, Injustice and the Welfare State: Part 1. An Ombudsman for the Poor?" *The Nation*, February 28, 1966.

Coe, Rodney. "Self Conception and Institutionalization." In Arnold Rose and Warren Peterson, eds., *Older People and Their Social World*. Philadelphia: F. A. Davis, 1965.

Cohen, Neil P. "The English Board of Visitors: Lay Outsiders as

Inspectors and Decision Makers in Prisons." *Federal Probation* (December 1976), vol. 40, no. 4.

Connecticut Nursing Home Ombudsman Office. "Annual Report." Hartford, Conn.: Connecticut Department on Aging, 1979.

Connecticut, State of. "An Act Creating a Nursing Home Ombudsman Office." Substitute House Bill No. 8037, Public Act No. 77-575.

Cromwell, Paul F., Jr. "A Vote for the Jail Ombudsman." *Federal Probation* (March 1974), vol. 38, no. 1.

Daley, R. M. and D. T. Jost. "The Nursing Home Reform Act of 1979." *Illinois Bar Journal* (1980), vol. 68.

Danet, Brenda. "Toward a Method to Evaluate the Ombudsman Role." *Administration and Society* (November 1978), vol. 10, no. 3.

Danet, Brenda and Harriet Hartman. "Coping with Bureaucracy: The Israeli Case." *Social Forces* (September 1972), vol. 51, no. 1.

Davidoff, Paul. "Advocacy and Pluralism in Planning." *Journal of the American Institute of Planners* (November 1965), vol. 31, no. 4.

Decker, Barry and Paul Bonner, eds. *PSRO: Organization for Regional Peer Review.* Cambridge, Mass.: Ballinger Publishing, 1973.

Delany, Carol A. and Kathleen A. Davies. *Nursing Home Ombudsman Project Final Report: The Pennsylvania Experience.* Harrisburg, Pa.: Pennsylvania Advocates for Better Care, 1979.

Dolan, Paul. "Pseudo-Ombudsman." *National Civic Review* (July 1969), vol. 69, no. 7.

Donabedian, Avedis. *The Definition of Quality and Approaches to Its Assessment.* Ann Arbor, Mich.: Health Administration Press, 1980.

—— "Evaluating the Quality of Medical Care." *Milbank Memorial Fund Quarterly* (July 1977), vol. 44, no. 3 (Part 2).

Eckert, Dorothy. "Advocacy in the Context of the Sociology of Knowledge: The Efficacy of the Ombudsman in the Health (Illness) Care Delivery System." Dissertation, Wayne State University, 1976.

Eggert, Gerald M. et al. "Caring for the Patient with Long Term Disability." *Geriatrics* (October 1977), vol. 32, no. 10.

Ettlinger, Roy A. "Advocate Informs Patients of Rights and Responsibilities." *Hospital & Community Psychiatry* (July 1973), vol. 24, no. 7.

Etzioni, Amitai. "The Third Sector and Domestic Missions." *Public Administration Review* (July/August 1973), vol. 33, no. 4.

Fay, John J., Jr. "Annual Report of the Ombudsman for the Institutionalized Elderly." Trenton, N.J.: Office of the Ombudsman for the Institutionalized Elderly, 1979.

Federal Council on the Aging, DHHS. "The Need for Long Term Care: Information and Issues." DHHS Publication 81-20704. Washington, D.C.: Office of Human Development Services, U.S. Government Printing Office, 1981.

Felton, Gary S. et al. "New Roles for New Professional Mental Health Workers. *Community Mental Health Journal* (Spring 1974), vol. 10, no. 1.

Ferguson, Vashtye and Ann Tydeman. "Organizing Around Nursing Home Issues." Washington, D.C.: National Citizens' Coalition for Nursing Home Reform, n.d.

Fitzharris, Timothy L. *The Desirability of a Correctional Ombudsman.* Berkeley: Institute of Governmental Studies, University of California, 1973.

Florida, State of. Adult Congregate Living Facilities Act of 1975, ch. 75-233 (as amended by ch. 77-401). Reported in State of Florida, *Annual Report of the Nursing Home Ombudsman Committee.* Tallahassee, Fla.: State Nursing Home Ombudsman Committee, 1979.

—— *Annual Report of the Nursing Home Ombudsman Committee.* Tallahassee, Fla.: State Nursing Home Ombudsman Committee, 1978.

—— *Annual Report of the Nursing Home Ombudsman Committee.* Tallahassee, Fla.: State Nursing Home Ombudsman Committee, 1979.

—— *Annual Report of the Long Term Care Ombudsman Committee.* Tallahassee, Fla.: State Long Term Care Ombudsman Committee, 1980.

—— *Annual Report of the Long Term Care Ombudsman Committee.* Brooksville, Fla.: State Long Term Care Ombudsman Committee, 1981.

Forman, Allen. "The Nursing Home Ombudsman Demonstration Program." *Health Services Reports* (March/April 1974), vol. 89, no. 2.

Fox, Raymond. "The Ombudsman: A Process Model for Humanizing Accountability." *Administration in Social Work* (Summer 1981), vol. 5, no. 2.

Freidson, Eliot. "Dominant Professions, Bureaucracy and Client Services." In Yeheskel Hasenfeld and Richard English, eds., *Human Service Organizations.* Ann Arbor: University of Michigan Press, 1977.

Friedmann, Karl. "The Public and the Ombudsman: Perceptions and

Attitudes in Britain and in Alberta." *Canadian Journal of Political Science* (September 1977), vol. 10, no. 3.

Gellhorn, Walter. *Ombudsmen and Others: Citizens' Protectors in Nine Countries.* Cambridge, Mass.: Harvard University Press, 1967.

George, Linda K. *Quality of Care in Nursing Homes: Attitudinal and Environmental Factors.* Durham, N.C.: Duke University, 1979.

Gilbert, Neil and Harry Specht. "Advocacy and Professional Ethics." *Social Work* (July 1976), vol. 21, no. 4.

Gosfield, Alice. *PSRO's: The Law and the Health Consumer.* Cambridge, Mass.: Ballinger Publishing, 1975.

Gottesman, Leonard E. and Norman C. Bourestom. "Why Nursing Homes Do What They Do." *The Gerontologist* (December 1974), vol. 14, no. 6.

Grafton, C. L. and M. A. Rivera. "Student Perceptions of the Ombudsman's Role in a Community College." *College Student Journal* (1976), vol. 10, no. 4.

Grosser, Charles. "Community Development Programs Serving the Urban Poor." *Social Work* (July 1965), vol. 10, no. 3.

—— "A Polemic on Advocacy." In Alfred J. Kahn, ed., *Shaping the New Social Work.* New York: Columbia University Press, 1973.

—— *New Directions in Community Organization: From Enabling to Advocacy.* New York: Praeger Publishers, 1976.

Gustafson, D. et al. "Measuring the Quality of Care in Nursing Homes: A Pilot Study in Wisconsin." *Public Health Reports* (July–August 1980), vol. 95, no. 4.

Gwyn, William B. *Barriers to Establishing Urban Ombudsmen: The Case of Newark.* Berkeley: Institute of Governmental Studies, University of California, 1974.

—— "The British PCA: Ombudsman or Ombudsmouse?" *Journal of Politics* (February 1973), vol. 35, no. 1.

Harvey, Judith W. "Comment on What a University Ombudsman Does." *Journal of Higher Education* (January/February 1978), vol. 49, no. 1.

Haug, Marie. "Doctor Patient Relationships and the Older Patient." *Journal of Gerontology* (November 1979), vol. 34, no. 6.

Hazard, Geoffry C. "The Ombudsman: Quasi-Legal and Legal Representation in Public Assistance Administration." In Thomas Sherrard, ed., *Social Welfare and Urban Problems.* New York: Columbia University Press, 1968.

Henry, Jules. *Culture Against Man.* New York: Random House, 1963.

Hill, Larry B. "The New Zealand Ombudsman's Authority System." *Political Science* (July 1968), vol. 20, no. 1.

—— "Institutionalization, the Ombudsman and Bureaucracy." *American Political Science Review* (September 1974), vol. 68, no. 3.

—— *The Model Ombudsman: Institutionalizing New Zealand's Democratic Experiment.* Princeton, N.J.: Princeton University Press, 1976.

—— *Ombudsmen, Bureaucracy, and Democracy.* New York: Oxford University Press, 1975.

Howard, John B. and Kenneth E. Strong. "Evaluating the Quality of Nursing Home Care." *Journal of the American Geriatrics Society* (November 1977), vol. 25, no. 11.

Hunter, Sylvia. "A Plan for a New York State Nursing Home Patient Ombudsman Program." New York: Community Council of Greater New York, 1977.

Huttmann, Barbara. *The Patient's Advocate: The Complete Handbook of Patients' Rights.* New York: Penguin Books, 1981.

Jordan, Vernon. "Voluntarism in America." *Vital Speeches,* June 1, 1977.

Kahana, Eva. "Matching Environments to Needs of the Aged: A Conceptual Scheme." In Jaber F. Gubrium, ed., *Late Life: Recent Developments in the Sociology of Aging.* Springfield, Ill.: Charles C. Thomas, 1975.

Kahn, Kenneth A. et al. "A Multidisciplinary Approach to Assessing the Quality of Care in Long-Term Care Facilities." *The Gerontologist* (February 1977), vol. 17, no. 1.

Katz, George C. "Advocacy in a Total Institution: The Making of an Ombudsman." *American Journal of Orthopsychiatry* (March 1971), vol. 41, no. 2.

Kauffman, B. K. and G. M. Boyle. "Family Advisory Councils in the Long Term Care Facility." In *Proceedings of the Fifth North American Symposium on Long Term Care Administration.* Washington, D.C.: American College of Nursing Home Administrators, 1979.

Kayser-Jones, Jeanie S. *Old, Alone and Neglected: Care of the Aged in Scotland and the United States.* Berkeley: University of California Press, 1981.

King County [Washington] Coalition of Nursing Home Resident Councils. *The Bulletin,* April 1981.

Koltveit, Thomas H. "Counselor-Consultant as Quasi-Ombudsman." *Personnel and Guidance Journal* (November 1973), vol. 52, no. 3.

Kopolow, Louis E. "Meeting the Patients' Rights Challenge through

Mental Health Advocacy." *Hospital & Community Psychiatry* (May 1977), vol. 28, no. 5.

Kosberg, Jordan I. "Making Institutions Accountable: Research and Policy Issues." *The Gerontologist* (December 1974), vol. 14, no. 6.

Kosberg, Jordan I. and Sheldon S. Tobin. "Variability Among Nursing Homes." *The Gerontologist* (Autumn 1972), vol. 12, no. 3.

Laking, G. R. "The Ombudsman and Medicine." *New Zealand Medical Journal* (November 1978), vol. 88, no. 624.

Langton, Stuart. "The New Voluntarism." *Journal of Voluntary Action Research* (January/March 1981), vol. 10, no. 1.

Langton, Stuart, ed. *Citizen Participation in America.* Lexington, Mass.: Lexington Books, D. C. Heath, 1978.

Larson, A. William. *Ed-Om: A Comprehensive Approach to Institutional Justice in Education,* Perspective Series No. 7, n.d.

Lieberman, Morton, Sheldon S. Tobin, and Darrell Slover. "The Effects of Relocation on Long Term Geriatric Patients." Final report to the Department of Mental Health, State of Illinois, Project #17-328, 1968.

Linn, Margaret W., Lee Gurel, and Bernard S. Linn. "Patient Outcomes as a Measure of Quality of Nursing Home Care." *American Journal of Public Health* (April 1977), vol. 67, no. 4.

Linnane, Patrick. *Ombudsman for Nursing Homes: Structure and Process.* DHEW Publication No. (OHD) 78-20293. Washington, D.C.: U.S. Government Printing Office, 1977.

Loeser, William D. et al. "Federal Regulation of Medical Practice in Nursing Homes." *Forum on Medicine* (August 1980), vol. 3, no. 8.

Love, Margaret and Molly Rechnitzer. "Patient Rights and the Elderly." Paper presented at the 34th Annual Scientific Meeting of the Gerontological Society of America, Toronto, Canada, 1981.

Lowi, Theodore J. *The End of Liberalism: Ideology, Policy, and the Crisis of Public Authority.* New York: Norton, 1969.

Luke, Roice D. and R. Wayne Boss. "Barriers Limiting the Implementation of Quality Assurance Programs." *Health Services Research* (Fall 1981), vol. 16, no. 3.

McGowan, Brenda. *Case Advocacy: A Study of the Interventive Process in Child Advocacy.* New York: Columbia University School of Social Work, 1973.

Madison, Terry M. "Those Who Speak Up." *Mental Health* (National Association for Mental Health), (1975), vol. 59, no. 2.

Mailick, Mildred D. "Patient Representative Programs in Short Term

General Hospitals and Their Relation to Social Work." Dissertation, Columbia University, 1978.

Mallory, Bruce L. "The Ombudsman in a Residential Institution: A Description of the Role and Suggested Training Areas." *Mental Retardation* (October 1977), vol. 15, no. 5.

Massachusetts Department of Elder Affairs. "Massachusetts Older Americans Advocacy Assistance Program Semi-Annual Report." Boston: Department of Elder Affairs, 1979.

Milliken, Robert and Ted R. Urich. "The Community Ombudsman: Program for Parent-Child Advocacy." *NASSP Bulletin*, October 1976.

Moore, John E. "Ombudsman and the Ghetto." *Connecticut Law Review* (December 1968), vol. 1, no. 2.

Moss, Frank E. and Val J. Halmandaris. *Too Old, Too Sick, Too Bad.* Germantown, Md.: Aspen Systems, 1979.

Nancoo, Stephen. "Administrative Theory and Bureaucratic Control: A Study of the Ombudsman Idea in Trinidad and Tobago." *Indian Journal of Public Administration* (April–June 1977), vol. 23, no. 2.

National Center for Health Statistics. "Current Estimates from the Health Interview Survey, United States, 1978." *Vital and Health Statistics*, Series 13 (130). DHEW Publication No. (PHS) 80-1551, Public Health Service. Washington, D.C.: U.S. Government Printing Office, 1979.

National Center for Health Statistics and Esther Hing. "Nursing Home Residents: Utilization, Health Status and Care Received, 1977 National Nursing Home Survey." *Vital and Health Statistics*, Series 13, No. 51. DHHS Publication No. (PHS) 81-1712, Public Health Service. Washington, D.C.: U.S. Government Printing Office, 1977.

National Citizens' Coalition for Nursing Home Reform. "A Report on 1980 State Nursing Home Legislation." Washington, D.C.: National Citizens' Coalition for Nursing Home Reform, 1980.

—— "A Report on the White House Mini-Conference on the Rights of the Institutionalized Elderly and the Role of the Volunteer." Washington, D.C.: National Citizens' Coalition for Nursing Home Reform, 1981.

—— "State Nursing Home Legislative Update." Washington, D.C.: National Citizens' Coalition for Nursing Home Reform, 1981.

Nelson, David and Kenneth Starck. "The Newspaper Ombudsman as Viewed by the Rest of the Staff." *Journalism Quarterly* (Autumn 1974), vol. 51, no. 3.

Neugarten, Bernice L. "The Future and the Young-Old." *The Gerontologist* (February 1975), vol. 15, no. 1 (Supplement).

Newmark, Louis. "The Development of a Residents' Council in a Home for the Aged." *The Gerontologist* (March 1963), vol. 3, no. 1.

New York City Nursing Home Patient Ombudsman Program. "Outline of Nursing Home Patient Interaction with Long Term Care Facilities." New York: the Program, n.d.

New York City Nursing Home Patient Ombudsman Program. *OmbudsNews* (February 1980), vol. 2, no. 2.

New York State Commission on Quality of Care for the Mentally Disabled. "Boards of Visitors: A Basic Orientation." New York: the Commission, 1980.

New York State Moreland Act Commission on Nursing Homes and Residential Facilities. *Regulating Nursing Home Care: The Paper Tigers.* New York: the Commission, 1975.

New York State Office for the Aging, Nursing Home Patient Ombudsman Program. "New York State Office for the Aging Nursing Home Patient Ombudsman Program, First Annual Report, October 1, 1977–September 30, 1978." New York: Office for the Aging, 1979.

New York *Times.* July 15, 1982.

Northey, J. F. "New Zealand's Parliamentary Commissioner." In Donald C. Rowat, ed., *The Ombudsman: Citizen's Defender.* London: George Allen and Unwin, Ltd., 1965.

Nursing Home Interests Section, Administration on Aging. "The Nursing Home Ombudsman Demonstration Program." Mimeo; 1975.

O'Connell, Brian. "From Service to Advocacy to Empowerment." *Social Casework* (April 1978), vol. 59, no. 4.

"Older Americans Advocacy Assistance Program." Mimeo; n.d.

Park, Clara and Leon Shapiro. "Being Your Child's Ombudsman at School and Elsewhere." *Exceptional Parent,* August 1976.

Parker, Pamela and Vicky Shields. *Resident Council Resource Kit.* Minneapolis: Nursing Home Residents' Advisory Council, 1981.

Parsons, Talcott. "The Sick Role and Role of the Physician Reconsidered." *Milbank Memorial Fund Quarterly* (Summer 1975), vol. 53, no. 3.

Pateman, Carole. *Participation and Democratic Theory.* London: Cambridge University Press, 1970.

Payne, James E. "Ombudsman Roles for Social Workers." *Social Work* (January 1972), vol. 17, no. 1.

Penn, Arthur. "Advocate from Within." *Trial* (February 1976), vol. 12, no. 2.

Pincus, Allen. "Toward a Conceptual Framework for Studying Institutional Environments in Homes for the Aged." Dissertation, University of Wisconsin, 1968.

Pincus, Allen and Vivian Wood. "Methodological Issues in Measuring the Environment in Institutions for the Aged and Its Impact on Residents." *Aging and Human Development* (May 1970), vol. 1, no. 2.

Pletcher, Philip. "The Curriculum Ombudsman: A Potentially Relevant Medical School Role." *Journal of Medical Education* (January 1974), vol. 49, no. 1.

Pugh, Sir Idwal. "On Being an Ombudsman." *Social Policy and Administration* (Spring 1980), vol. 14, no. 1.

Reeder, Leo G. "The Patient-Client as a Consumer: Some Observations on the Changing Professional Client Relationship." *Journal of Health and Social Behavior* (December 1972), vol. 13, no. 4.

Regan, John J. "Quality Assurance Systems in Nursing Homes." *Journal of Urban Law* (Fall 1975), vol. 53, no. 2.

—— "When Nursing Home Patients Complain: The Ombudsman or the Patient Advocate." *Georgetown Law Journal* (February 1977), vol. 65, no. 3.

Robb, Susanne et al. "Advocacy for the Aged." *American Journal of Nursing* (October 1979), vol. 79, no. 10.

Robinson, G. Erlick and Naomi Alboim. "The Use of Non-professional Change Agents in an Institution." *Canadian Psychiatric Association Journal* (1974), vol. 19, no. 5.

Rowat, Donald C., ed. *The Ombudsman: Citizen's Defender.* London: George Allen and Unwin, Ltd., 1965; 2d ed., 1968.

Sandler, Ake. "An Ombudsman for the United States." *The Annals of the American Academy of Political and Social Science* (May 1968), vol. 377.

Shore, Herbert. "Try a Residents' Council." *Professional Nursing Home* (November 1964).

Silverbank, Francine. "Role Perceptions of the Ombudsman." *Intellect* (January 1974), vol. 5, no. 102.

Silverstone, Barbara. *Establishing Resident Councils.* New York: Federation of Protestant Welfare Agencies, Division on Aging, 1974.

—— "Expert vs. Consumer Viewpoints: An Organizational Analysis of the Contrasts in Descriptions of Homes for the Aged by Administrators and Indigenous Residents." Dissertation, Columbia University, 1973.

Smith, Eleanor and Pauline Winnick. "Your Library: Neighborhood Ombudsman." *American Education* (November 1976), vol. 12, no. 9.

Sosin, Michael. "Social Work Advocacy and the Implementation of Legal Mandates." *Social Casework: The Journal of Contemporary Social Work* (May 1979), vol. 60, no. 5.

Stacey, Frank. *Ombudsmen Compared.* Oxford: Clarendon Press, 1978.

Stannard, Charles I. "Old Folks and Dirty Work: The Social Conditions for Patient Abuse in a Nursing Home." *Social Problems* (Winter 1973), vol. 20, no. 3.

Stewart, Kenneth L. "What a University Ombudsman Does." *Journal of Higher Education* (January/February 1978), vol. 49, no. 1.

Strahan, Genevieve. "Inpatient Health Facilities Statistics, United States, 1978." *Vital and Health Statistics: Data from the National Health Survey* (1981), vol. 14, no. 24.

Sullivan, Ellen Wahl. *Corrective Mechanisms for Resolving Abuses and Upgrading Care in Institutions for the Aged.* New York: Center for Policy Research, 1979.

Sundram, Clarence J. "Independent Oversight of Mental Hygiene Facilities: The New York Experience." *Journal of Psychiatric Treatment and Evaluation* (1980), vol. 2, no. 1.

Tibbles, Lance. "Ombudsman for American Prisons," *North Dakota Law Review* (1972), vol. 48.

Trueblood, Ann and Gary Anderson. "Nursing Home Ombudsmen Involvement with Resident Governance in Homes for the Aging." Washington, D.C.: American Association of Homes for the Aging, 1981.

Tydeman, Ann. "Putting the Pieces Together: A Guide to Coalition Building." Washington, D.C.: National Citizens' Coalition for Nursing Home Reform, n.d.

U.S. Department of Commerce, Bureau of the Census. *Current Population Reports, Special Studies.* Series P-23, No. 59. Second printing (rev.), January 1978. *Demographic Aspects of Aging and the Older Population in the United States.* Washington, D.C.: U.S. Government Printing Office, 1978.

U.S. Government. *Federal Register,* March 31, 1980.

Verkuil, Paul R. "The Ombudsman and the Limits of the Adversary System." *Columbia Law Review* (May 1975), vol. 75, no. 4.

Vladeck, Bruce C. *Unloving Care: The Nursing Home Tragedy.* New York: Basic Books, 1980.

Vosburgh, William W. "Client Rights, Advocacy and Volunteerism." *Journal of Voluntary Action Research* (January/March 1981), vol. 10, no. 1.

Vosburgh, William W. and Drew Hyman. "Advocacy and Bureaucracy: The Life and Times of a Decentralized Citizens' Advocacy Program." *Administrative Science Quarterly* (December 1973), vol. 18, no. 4.

Weatherby, Roberta G. "Regulation of Nursing Homes: Adequate Protection for the Nation's Elderly?" *St. Mary's Law Journal* (1976), vol. 8, no. 2.

Wildavsky, Aaron. *Speaking Truth to Power: The Art and Craft of Policy Analysis.* Boston: Little, Brown, 1979.

Williams, Theartrice. "Between the Keepers and the Kept." *Trial* (March 1976), vol. 12, no. 3.

—— "The Minnesota Corrections Ombudsman." *Social Work* (November 1975), vol. 20, no. 6.

Wilson, Sally Hart. "Nursing Home Patient's Rights: Are They Enforceable?" *The Gerontologist* (June 1978), vol. 18, no. 3.

Wolfensberger, W. et al. *The Principle of Normalization in Human Services.* Toronto, Ontario, Canada: National Institute of Mental Retardation, 1972.

Wolkon, George H. and Sharon Moriwaki. "The Ombudsman: A Serendipitous Mental Health Intervention." *Community Mental Health Journal* (Fall 1977), vol. 13, no. 3.

Wyner, Alan J., ed. *Executive Ombudsmen in the United States.* Berkeley: Institute of Governmental Studies, University of California, 1973.

Zweig, Franklin M. "The Social Worker as Legislative Ombudsman." *Social Work* (January 1969), vol. 14, no. 1.

NAME INDEX

GENERAL INDEX

The Social Work and Social Issues Series

The Columbia University School of Social Work publication series, Social Work and Social Issues, is concerned with the implications of social work practice and social welfare policy for solving problems. Each volume is an independent work. The series is intended to contribute to the knowledge base of social work education, to facilitate communication with related disciplines, and to serve as a background for public policy discussion. Books in the series are:

Shirley Jenkins, editor. *Social Security in International Perspective* 1969.
George Brager and Harry Specht. *Community Organizing.* 1973.
Alfred J. Kahn, editor. *Shaping the New Social Work.* 1973.
Shirley Jenkins and Elaine Norman. *Beyond Placement.* 1975.
Deborah Shapiro. *Agencies and Foster Children.* 1975.
David Fanshel and Eugene B. Shinn. *Children in Foster Care.* 1978.
Carol Meyer, editor. *Clinical Social Work in the Eco-Systems Perspective.* 1983.
Abraham Monk, Lenard W. Kaye, and Howard Litwin. *Resolving Grievances in the Nursing Home.* 1984.